Belief to HEAL

Mastering the Mindset to Heal

Matt Rowe

Copyright © 2022 by IDENTITY OF HEALTH PUBLISHING. All rights reserved.

No part of this publication may be reproduced, stored in a retrieval system, or transmitted in any form or by any means, electronic, mechanical, photocopying, recording, scanning, or otherwise, without the prior written permission of the author.

Limit of Liability/Disclaimer of Warranty: This publication is designed to provide accurate and authoritative information in regard to the subject matter covered. It is sold with the understanding that neither the author nor the publisher is engaged in rendering legal, medical, psychological, or other professional services. While the publisher and author have used their best efforts in preparing this book, they make no representations or warranties with respect to the accuracy or completeness of the contents of this book and specifically disclaim any implied warranties of merchantability or fitness for a particular purpose. No warranty may be created or extended by sales representatives or written sales materials. The advice contained herein may not be suitable for your situation. You should consult with a professional when appropriate. Neither the publisher nor the author shall be liable for any loss of profit or any other commercial damages, including but not limited to special, incidental, consequential, personal, or other damages.

BELIEF TO HEAL: Mastering the Mindset to Heal
By Matthew Rowe

Hardcover: 979-8-9860404-1-7
Paperback: 979-8-9860404-2-4
ebook: 979-8-9860404-3-1
Audio book: 979-8-9860404-0-0

Cover and interior design by Heidi Sutherlin at My Creative Pursuits
Edited by Cortni L. Merritt at SRD Editing Services

Printed in the United States of America

IDENTITY OF HEALTH PUBLISHING
Denver, Colorado, U.S.A.

Dedication

For Henry and Alex. You are my reason, my purpose, and my true loves. Thank you for sharing this incredible life with me.

Acknowledgments

Writing this book stretched every belief I had in myself to continue and complete what you read today. None of this would have been possible without my best friend and love, Dixie Willis. You encouraged and believed in me when I felt alone, and you challenged me to believe and see what I could not. I am blessed to be with you and love you. Thank you for finding me again, in this lifetime.

I'm eternally grateful to my kids, Henry and Alex, who challenge me every day to be a better man. My reasons to heal. I love being a part of your beautiful lives. Thank you for the lessons you taught me, the love you poured on me, and the experiences of life I share with you. I also want to thank my parents, Jennifer and Tom, and sisters, Becky, Kate, and Kim, who were my teachers and tough-love givers in life. I would not be who I am today without the lessons and love you gave me. Thank you for believing in me through all my abrupt changes and times when I pushed you away.

To my editor, Cortni Merritt. I believe the right teachers come into our lives at the right time and when we are open to receiving them. This book would not be, if it were not for your wisdom. You helped me realize that I am an author. You were patient when I went dark during my divorce and provided structure and guidance when I had no idea where to take a step. You have a gift, and thank you for sharing it with me and being a part of publishing this book.

Although these periods of my life were filled with many ups and downs, my friends became the rocks along the way. Every step had its own purpose, and I want to thank you for being with me. From my friend Mike in college, who taught me how to play guitar and introduced me to a bigger way of being with books of spiritual living, to Greg, who I will always see as a brother who showers me with praise and grounds me to my true Self. Thank you for being in my life.

Writing a book about the story of your life is a surreal process. I'm forever indebted to my teachers and guides: Anthony William, Michael Singer, Bruce Lipton, Mitch Albom, Deepak Chopra, Louise Hay, Gregg Braden, Dr. Joe Dispenza, Wayne Dyer, and Roger Teel, along with many others. It is because of your efforts and encouragement that I have a legacy to pass on to my family, where one didn't exist before. You are all part of my healing team. Also, to all my clients who provided breadcrumbs of encouragement along my path.

Finally, to God and my Oneness with You, and to the right people, places, and events that made this book possible.

Contents

Introduction 1
Central Terms & Concepts 7
Chapter 1: My Backstory 11
Chapter 2: Becoming Aware 27
Chapter 3: Letting Go 45
Chapter 4: Envisioning Something New & Support 57
Chapter 5: Who are You? 71
Chapter 6: What Do You Want? 85
Chapter 7: Getting Out of Your Own Way/Un-Learning the Past/Opening Mindset to Healing 97
Chapter 8: Mindset to Heal 115
Chapter 9: Healing Behaviors 129
Chapter 10: Healed/New Identity 141
Chapter 11: Small Steps/The Essential Nature of all Progress 149
Chapter 12: The Importance of Belief 159
Chapter 13: Living without Fear 169
Chapter 14: Inspiring Others 179
Chapter 15: Conclusion 185
References 189
About Author Matt Rowe 197

Introduction

A New Reality

When we are diagnosed with a disease or left with a life-altering injury, the fear can become overwhelming. We attempt to keep our chin up as our world crashes around us. Who We Think We Are—with our hopes, ambitions, and dreams—is taken away in a breath and shaken with every doctor's appointment. We are not always told a positive prognosis; we sometimes are given the worst-case scenario, protecting the doctor and leaving us feeling lost with little belief that it will get better. We are prescribed medications that have side effects and given injections or surgeries that mask the pain.

What if it did not have to be this way?

Our disease or injury gives us an opportunity to see past the egoic nature of life, making us aware of what is truly important. Although material desires may be important, we make it our everything, leaving us with the stress of an impossible dream of "enough." We may fight to return to the lives we once had, as we beg and plead for God, the Universe, or Source to bring it back to us.

It is at this moment, we have two roads we can walk down: a path of frustration, blame, and anger, which only brings more of the same, or we can walk the path of love, joy, acceptance, and surrender to what is truly important—*YOU*. As we realize that there is another way, our eyes open to the possibility that our disease is acting *for* us, to wake us up, rather than acting *to* us.

As we wake up to ourselves, we begin to see answers and begin listening to and hearing about new ways to heal. Along with doctors, we build a life of possibility, and we begin to Believe and know ourselves at a deeper level.

My Mission of Hope

We are told solutions that leave us with a myopic view of our disease or injury. I see a problem with the way society currently tells people to deal with a disease, injury, or chronic pain. Some injuries are easily addressed and fixed with a minor amount of life's disruptions, but what happens when these disruptions are life altering?

I believe that chemistry might help us live better, in some ways. There is some chemistry and science that heals disease, and there are surgeries that are miracles, but what happens when these options are not available for you and you are left with a "wait-and-see" approach?

When we leave a doctor's office, where they tell us a diagnosis/ prognosis, we begin to think about our past and all the things we can't do that we could before. We have our routines and habits that led us to this point, and with the blink of an eye, they all change. We may begin to blame ourselves as we go through the stages of loss that may leave us feeling like we are not enough. The shame and guilt of what happened may creep in, and this adds gasoline to an already large blaze of negativity and scarcity.

Leaving a doctor's office with life-changing news can be a brutal reality. We are told that remaining positive, altering our diets, avoiding toxins, and reducing stress are helpful suggestions, but we are not told *how*, nor are we supported to explore these alternative ways. The mainstream media is more concerned with a "magic pill" with more possible side effects than with hope. At this moment, we have an opportunity to explore and practice food as medicine, positive thought, and stress-reduction techniques, while creating a new sense of being.

We discover *ourselves* on this journey; we discover how amazing our lives are and what is important. This awe and amazement of our own powerful selves has us adopting the powerful nature of Self-love and the Belief that we will get better.

This Belief turns into knowing that what we do to heal from the inside out is giving us control, as we listen to inspired suggestions and thoughts. We take action on understanding better how the natural chemistries of food and exercise work within the human body.

> We begin to realize how amazing our
> bodies are to heal disease and injury,
> if we allow ourselves the patience,
> Belief, and understanding to do so.

My Reason for Awareness

In the winter of 2008, after being an All-American Triathlete, I paralyzed my right leg from the waist down. After healing my leg with surgery, my Belief and desire had me finishing Ironman, in 2011. Instead of paying attention to *why* this injury happened, I continued with the egoic desire of more and was left with stress, anger, and twenty-five to thirty strokes per day. Left with little understanding or reason, I delved into food as medicine and reversed the strokes I was experiencing.

Once again, instead of dealing with the stress and feelings of not being "enough," I ignored what was important, until being diagnosed with multiple sclerosis in 2017. That is when I woke up.

I began exploring what is important, and I began loving myself enough to slow down. I studied meditation practices and medicinal properties of food, as I reduced my oxidative stress. As I discovered practices that left me feeling better and increasing my knowledge, I found myself studying body chemistry and mindfulness practices and working to understand the toxins in our food and water. As I made choices—using myself as the test subject—I began to feel better and regain my life.

I found myself waking up each morning with a new sense of hope and a belief that my life was going to be better, always attracting the opportunities and people to enhance this belief. There is knowledge and research on the specifics, but without the Belief that they will work, they rarely do, or the solutions are revealed as a Band-Aid, used to mask the real reason. It is not until we make the choice to step beyond the research and step into the essence of our beautiful selves that we understand and believe that our choices are right.

My Intent & Desire

Who We Think We Are and *What We Want* lead to our behaviors. I did not know at the time, but I was leveraging my identity and mindset.

What happens when our lives have been abruptly changed due to a disease or injury? The story of my athletic and weight loss changes sound great and logical, but the difficult part comes when we mix fear into this equation. Fear can lead to negative thoughts, which lead to statements of the past—like "I used to," "I shouldn't," "I can't anymore." These thoughts can lead to behaviors of depression, due to not being who you once thought you were.

Our depression can lead us to stress, and our stress is known to cause disease. If we all learned how to eat better, we could eradicate disease entirely, once and for all. Of course, that might take more than a single generation putting forth a ton of effort into understanding human nature and our interactive biochemistry with the world around us. But, as crazy as it sounds, I think if everyone put in 100 percent effort toward what is truly important, instead of relying on the answers and prescriptions of someone else, we could begin to heal.

During my journey, I became a health coach, meditation practitioner, and Reiki master; I am still doing CrossFit (not in a wheelchair), and I was driven to help others heal. In its own sick way, my disease has been the greatest gift ever handed to me.

During all my experiences, I learned that:

- Food is medicine
- Dangerous toxins exist in our food and environment, and I learned how to avoid them
- I *am* enough

- To slow down
- To stop taking myself so seriously
- To laugh
- To love myself
- To trust myself

After removing toxins from my diet and flooding my body with nutrients, I began to feel better. Instead of being forced to use a wheelchair, within seven months of diagnosis, like my doctor promised, I actually began to feel better than expected, much like I used to before the injuries. At that point, I was even more convinced and determined to halt and reverse MS.

Why Should You Keep Reading

This book is for anyone who has ever experienced an ongoing painful situation. It's for anyone who's ever received an unexpected medical diagnosis and for the loved ones and caregivers of people who receive such medical diagnoses. It's for anyone who's ever lost someone to chronic pain, and it's for anyone who's ever experienced anxiety and fear as a result of chronic pain.

It's for anyone who's tried other self-help books and meditation practices and not found relief. It's for anyone who loves food but hates memorizing health information. It's for someone who has wanted to take control of their health and find another way. It's for the person who is in the middle of following medical advice but looking for another way to help themselves, beyond what the doctors tell them.

> This book is for someone looking for the Belief, knowing that health is possible, no matter how difficult it may seem. It's for someone willing to remove all the blocks and do the hard work of discovering Who They Are.

Central Terms & Concepts

Awareness
"Awareness" (capitalized) throughout the text refers to **knowledgeable being—conscious, cognizant, informed,** and **alert living**. Awareness is the state or ability to perceive, to feel, or to be conscious of events, objects, or sensory patterns. Your Awareness dictates your responses and stress, based on various situations.

Belief
A (capitalized) "Belief" is an attitude that something *is* the case, or that some proposition about the world *is true*. The (lowercased) term "belief" refers to attitudes about the world that can be *either* true or false. To Believe something is to be convinced it is true; however, holding a belief does not require active introspection. Particular Beliefs can dictate actions, behavior, and events, making those Beliefs into truth or creating the physical representation of one's Belief.

Ego
In this text, the (capitalized) "Ego" is the psychological component of the personality represented by our conscious decision-making processes from the conscious and subconscious mind, which warn us of known danger or the potential dangers of an unknown situation, even if these potentialities are unfounded or untrue.

Fear
In the text, "fear" represents an intensely unpleasant emotion in response to perceiving or recognizing a danger or threat of change, which causes a stress response. Fear causes physiological changes that may produce behavioral reactions, such as mounting an aggressive response or fleeing from or avoiding the threat. Fear in human beings may occur in response to a certain stimulus based on past experiences, or in anticipation or expectation of a future threat, perceived as

a risk to oneself, especially due to change, confrontation, or the unknown. The common human response to fear is known as the "fight, flight, or freeze response."

Ideal Self
The Ideal Self is an idealized version of yourself created from what you have learned from your life experiences and the demands of society, combined with what you admire in your role models.

Identity
"Identity" encompasses the memories, experiences, relationships, and values that create one's sense of Self. This amalgamation creates a steady sense of Who You Are over time.

Inner Voice
Your "inner voice" is an "internal dialogue" or "inner monologue," "voice inside your head," or "inner voice." This voice can represent someone from your past, or it can represent your Self.

Intuition
Intuition is that identifiable sense of *knowing* what the right answer or decision is, even before you make it. It's a deep, internal, visceral feeling. You know your intuition is around when you say things like, "I can't really explain it, but..." or "It just felt right," or more likely, "It just felt wrong."

Mindset
Mindset is a set of Beliefs that shape how you make sense of the world and yourself. It influences how you think, feel, and behave in any given situation.

Perception
The process of taking in, choosing, organizing, and understanding sensory information. It includes collecting data from sense organs and interpreting this data based on past experiences, education, or current belief.

Present Moment
In the text, the (capitalized) "Present Moment" refers to this *specific moment in time*, which takes in feeling from the senses, the current situation, and the event.

Self vs. self
Self: There are two versions of the "self." The most common is the idea of our "self" made up of our personality characteristics, experiences, and daily interactions with others. This "self" is you as a person, a human. The more philosophical idea of "Self" is made up of our deeper core desires and is connected to our soul, spirit, or existence beyond the body and daily interactions with others. When I use (capitalized) "Self" in this book, I want you to think in terms of who you would be without your personality, experiences, and influence of others.

Self-esteem
Self-esteem is how we value and perceive ourselves, as physical beings. Self-esteem is based on opinions and (perhaps temporary) beliefs about ourselves, as people. Your self-esteem can affect whether you like and value your own Beliefs and opinions, and whether you are able to make decisions and assert yourself.

Self-image
Self-image is the personal view, or mental picture, that we have of ourselves. Self-image is a belief that describes the characteristics of the (human/physical) self, including personality characteristics like *intelligent*, *talented*, *selfish*, and *kind*, as well as physical characteristics like *beautiful*, *ugly*, *fat*, *brunette*, and *athletic*. However, a (capitalized) Self-image is the mental picture we have of our philosophical Self.

Support
In the text, "support" references a kind, empathetic, helpful person who understands your values and encourages you with loving accountability, assisting you with remaining on your journey during a difficult or unhappy time in your life.

Values

In the text, "Values" represent the core values, the fundamental Beliefs that a person consciously attempts to act in accordance with. These guiding principle Values dictate the person's behaviors, communications, and actions. Values are unique to each individual.

Who You Are

Throughout the text, (capitalized) Who You Are is defined as the core Values you see at the center of your Self-image. Although your external reality (house, car, job, spouse, social pressures, community, etc.) is important, these elements can easily be removed, and you would be left with the core Values that define Who You Are.

Chapter 1

My Backstory

> "Life is 10 percent what happens to you
> and 90 percent how you react to it."
>
> – Charles R. Swindoll, *The Grace Awakening*

My Story

As I began to heal, I adhered to the philosophies of the greatest thinker of the seventeenth century, René Descartes, even before I knew it. Descartes came to be known as the "father of the mind-body connection," and his best-known philosophy is "I think, therefore, I am."

Although, for me, I have found through experience that who I *thought* I was led to how I thought about myself, and this view of myself led to my behaviors, actions, and ultimately, the results I have experienced.

Descartes advised that a thinking person, in order to make the wisest decision possible, needed to review a situation from multiple angles, analyzing it from a series of perspectives, in order to reach the greatest and most accurate conclusion.

I have found that this is what I've had to do with my life. When injuries I could not predict changed the course of who I thought I was, when medical diagnoses I never anticipated altered the ways in which I interact with reality and myself, I could do nothing but adapt. And the best methods for adaptations were those that I found by looking at my situations with new, unique, and different-than-my-normal perspectives.

Of course, to understand my new and enhanced perspectives, we have to examine where I began. We must look over my previous understandings of the world. You must get to know a bit about who I used to be, and I'd like to show you what made me change so that you know that you, too, can change into who you'd like to become.

My Backstory—Childhood & Early Adolescence

I was the ruler of my neighborhood. Granted, I was only eight years old, but I can clearly remember that feeling of invincibility. As the sun peaked and showed its light, I was running out the door for the day. The neighborhood kids and I spent our days playing in the nearby creek, making ramps for bikes, and participating in games like "kick the can" or "ghost in the graveyard." I felt confident and unstoppable. I was truly living in the Present Moment. However, something changed drastically around the age of ten.

My self-assured and carefree persona was disrupted when my family moved only twenty miles away, which could have been one thousand miles for all I understood at that age. I entered a new school, with my unshakeable demeanor tested, and I struggled to maintain my young identity of a confident, popular kid.

Starting as the "new kid" at that age was quite difficult, especially while trying to develop new friendships. I was left feeling lost, and that's when I started to notice my inner critic, the little voice in the back of my head. This voice was with me day in and day out, commenting on everything I did. The voice became louder, and it was tearing me down every time I attempted to act with my prior confidence in my new setting. As a result, I began living my young life based on what I thought others wanted, and my feeling of invincibility began dissolving. The voice kept becoming louder and would say things like, "You can't", "What would someone else think?", "What if you fail?", or simply, "You are not good enough."

Over the years, my perceived failures and not being accepted began anchoring and solidifying who I thought I was. This overly persistent, negative voice began to impact how I viewed myself and the world around me. I went from feeling unstoppable to feeling like a lonely loser.

For a young, impressionable kid trying to find his way, this new identity of being fearful, lonely, overweight, and "unpopular" (in my mind) was starting to set in stone and become the belief of who I thought I was.

Through my young years, I developed a mask, altering who I was in order to receive the acceptance of others. I became enraptured by how others viewed me, and I tried multiple ways to change my self-perception. The whole time, I was letting go of myself and was trying to be anything and everything for those around me.

At this time, I made a good friend, Dan, and we both had a desire to be liked by girls. I remember many of our conversations revolved around skateboarding and girls, and we pursued them both as much as we could. Dan became a beacon of light for me as I was defining myself. Dan helped introduce me to girls and helped me become the "cool kid" I desperately wanted to be. Through this friendship, I was discovering *Who I Could Be*, and through that, I was finding my confidence again.

Backstory—High School & College

As I stepped into high school and college, I thought I could change my identity and be accepted with sports. Every day, I strapped on a figurative mask of what I thought others wanted to see.

In high school, I saw my older sister excel at everything she did academically. Her academic prowess—in my eyes—was a label I wanted, but I kept running into a roadblock: I disliked school. This dislike of school left me with Cs and Ds, while reinforcing my feeling of not being good enough.

I turned to sports, but that was difficult for an overweight kid. I tried wrestling and learned how to fail, over and over again. Through the failures of wrestling also came increased confidence; there is nothing like wearing a skin-tight outfit in front of others that helps you deal with any lack of confidence you may have. The rigors of the sport got me in shape, and I started to look and feel better about myself.

This sense of confidence must have done something, because I started to date girls and they were showing interest in me. I was learning about how to control my weight, and I found some joy in pushing myself. I soon started to experience the attention that I desired, when I injured myself. I did not intentionally seek to get injured but noticed it happening. I found myself pushing to extremes, pushing my body to the limits. My confidence started to show in all facets of my life, as the mask and persona I was showing everyone else became my primary focus, over grades or taking care of myself.

At this time in high school, I started to drink and party, as I strove to be the popular kid.

I sneaked into college with a low GPA. In college, I was not focused and was more in it for the experiences, not the education. At that time, I was feeling more confident but noticed the injuries did not lessen. During my freshman year of college, I joined rugby and discovered that a knee can most definitely be injured more than once, and the healing process takes longer than three months. I did not realize, at the time, that these injuries were a way to receive attention.

This pattern and identity of "not enough," although maturing with me, began to exhibit itself, as I tried to be the life of the party, in college. This route took me down some fun (and not so fun) adventures involving too much alcohol and marijuana and lots of risky choices. I pushed my body to the extreme because I was trying to impress everyone else, not staying true to or loving myself.

Backstory—Early Adult Life

After completing four years of college, getting married, and stepping into a career, I had little self-esteem, and it was obvious. My weight soon exceeded two hundred and fifty pounds, and that did not change until my wife became pregnant with our son. I decided that I was not going to die of a heart attack at age fifty, as doctors allude to if you are stressed out and overweight. I wanted to be there for my son when he needed me. Due to this strong reason to change, I began running and biking and developed new desires of how I wanted to live my life. Little did I know that this new athletic adventure was still masking my core need to be accepted.

With my new exercise regimen, I lost eighty-five pounds and began to shift my identity of being an overweight person. This gave me a small bit of confidence (even at eighty-five pounds lighter, I still viewed myself as a "fat" person). When I began running and biking, I found that I enjoyed it! Prior to my son being born, I signed up for my first race, and seven days after his birth, I won my age group in my first race.

I was hooked and began meeting other racers, who talked me into racing a triathlon, so I added swimming to the biking and running mix. After racing many multisport events over a four-year period, my confidence increased, as I became the person to beat. I wanted a label that people looked up to. I would push hard to win, no matter the pain. I did not care; I got the attention I desperately needed and wanted. This drive led me to earn an All-American Triathlete designation in triathlon at the half-Ironman distance and being the top of the field in most endurance events in my twenties and thirties.

> This was a great accomplishment,
> but I forgot something along the way: ME.

My training and habits became an obsession, and along with having a growing family, it became my focus and priority. Throughout these adventures and lessons, I thought that pushing myself harder and assuming the perfect persona or mask of what I thought others wanted was the answer. It felt good to finally feel better about myself, but it was all superficial. My outward persona was not only tricking those around me, but also myself.

Later on, I realized I was only hurting myself by pretending to have it all together. I had addressed part of what I wanted but never looked at who I was as a person, and I was left feeling angry, lost, and financially insecure; I was yelling at my kids and grabbing at any opportunity. I was miserable, and at one point, I even thought about ending it all permanently. This mindset and the mask I had developed led to the not-so-fun adventures that forced me to learn from life and finally discover Who I Was Meant to Be.

The Start of my Adult Journey—Ruptured Disc

Soon after earning my Honorable Mention as an All-American Triathlete, I was out shoveling snow, when one shovel full of heavy snow severely ruptured my L5 spinal disc. This left my right leg partially paralyzed, which meant I could no longer stand on my right tiptoes. Running was impossible, walking was difficult, and the injury was obvious to those around me, as I walked with a limp.

I was scared and avoided doctors, besides chiropractors, seeking advice from physical therapists who I considered friends. At that time, I heard horror stories of spinal disc fusions (removing the disc and having the bones on either side screwed together) from friends who had them done, only to find the discs on either side of the one repaired ruptured shortly after. I did everything I could to avoid having those types of serious conversations.

I believed there had to be another way, and I was not about to roll over and accept someone else's catastrophic opinion, no matter how qualified. I was most afraid of never being able to run, bike, or compete again. I was not ready or willing to change, so I tried to hide from the potential inevitable diagnosis and realization that I may have to address the inner critic who still plagued me.

With the avid determination to fix myself without destroying my triathlete identity, I tried plenty of unique treatments. I was pulled apart with traction to allow more space in my spine, with the hope that the message from my brain would reach my leg again.

Someone else used mirrors to try to play mental tricks on my brain to make me think my bad leg was functioning again. The experience of watching 90 percent of my muscle atrophy and leave my right leg was humbling. In May of 2008, I was approached by my medical team of chiropractors during yet another visit. They suggested surgery and said that I needed to meet with a neurologist.

I had lost 90 percent of the muscle in my right leg, and they were concerned that if I left the atrophy unaddressed, the leg could lose functionality, which would eventually end in amputation.

It was during this time that angels and teachers provided recommendations to a neurologist, who told me there was a 50 percent shot that a noninvasive surgery could fix my situation.

I remember being in the neurologist's office and asking him what my chances were of using my leg again. He clarified that the 50 percent odds were that I could improve, or he may paralyze me from the waist down. He would be working in an area very close to other areas important for lower limb functionality. The neurologist was proposing inserting a three-inch-long tube, about the width of your pinky finger, into my lower spine to allow instruments into the spinal area that would clean the scar tissue off the nerves that was created by the blown disc. Simple, right?

I explored the option of doing nothing and keeping with the chiropractic approach that was yielding zero functional improvements but leaving me happily pain-free. It became clear that if I did nothing, the leg would die, and I would have it amputated eventually—this was the only certainty. So, I went ahead with the surgery. Whether it was one leg amputated or both functionally gone due to paralysis, it felt like the same life sentence to me, and at least having the surgery gave me a 50 percent chance of doing what I loved again someday.

After Surgery

As I limped into the surgery center, all I could think about was how I wanted to run again. Just four months earlier, my journey of competing (and placing high on the leaderboards) in more than 100 multi-sport/running and cycling events had abruptly come to an end. Now, to be limping into a surgery center was a harsh and upsetting comparison, to say the least.

Fortunately, after the doctor spent two and a half hours painstakingly cleaning the damaged nerves, I physically walked out of the operation. I was now looking at a rehabilitation process that would take years. I was told that although the messages were now firing, the nerves were still severely damaged, and nerves only grow 1mm a day. If you do the math, I have a 31" inseam, which equals 787.4 mm and a twenty-six-month recovery. If I had decided "woe is me" and played the victim without holding onto hope, I do not believe I would have been open to calling the neurologist, listening to him, and moving forward with the surgery.

Rehab was not fun, realizing I had limitations. I went back to riding my bike and trying to run again. After a frustrating twenty-eight months of recovery, I did the only logical thing I could think of. On November 20, 2010, I signed up for Ironman Arizona. This made no sense; I had just bankrupted a company, had contemplated suicide, and was attempting to make my leg work again like it used to, which led to more frustration. I did not know where I was going to find the money to train, the drive to compete, and or a paying job to keep my family fed.

Unnoticed by me at the time, due to my long-lasting relationship with my inner critic, I was also telling myself all the ways it could not work.

My kids were what kept me moving forward, and we all agreed, although somewhat reluctantly, that I must finish Ironman (a 2.4-mile swim, a 112-mile bike ride, and a 26.2-mile run). I realized later, although it was never discussed or mentioned, that the only reason my family encouraged me to do this unthinkable feat was to preserve my mental health.

Ironman was going to take a great deal of dedication and training, and if this did not push me to recover to some semblance of my former self, then nothing would. At the time, I viewed it as an exciting challenge, but as I look back on it, it was much more than that. I needed a new identity, or at the very least, my old one back.

Being "an Ironman" had a nice ring to it, and on November 18, 2011, I overcame all the barriers and crossed the finish line in thirteen hours and twenty-four minutes.

TIAs & Meaning of Change

In one shovelful of snow, I went from the identity of being an honorable mention All–American Triathlete to someone who struggled to walk to his car.

Belief to Heal

After this event, I went back to fighting and getting the proverbial larger hammer to drive situations that were not working in my favor, as the anger, frustration, scarcity, and fear grew.

I was so afraid of going back to my pre-triathlon days, my past, and afraid to show the real me where I felt I was not enough.

After Ironman, the need to swim, bike, or run again was gone. That box had been checked, and I began to look for my next accomplishment.

It was at this time that a true friend who I consider like a brother kept talking about this incredible workout called CrossFit. I tried it and was immediately hooked, but the injuries and need to be accepted did not stop. During a particularly hard workout, which included box jumps (jumping onto a 24-inch-high wooden box), I happened to miss my mark on jump number eighty-nine, driving my shin into the side of the box. It was fortunate that I did not break my shin bone, but the scar still remains today. My treatment for the large gash I sustained included antibiotics—a lot of them—which extended over a three-month period. It was at this time I began to feel dizzy and tired, and my general mental well-being got progressively worse. What was happening to me?

I attributed my symptoms to stress, due to the pressure and high demands I was feeling at my workplace.

In January 2015, I visited a doctor again regarding the shin, and they prescribed me another round of antibiotics, this time more than 1500mg of Keflex. I did not question the doctors, because I had no reason to, at least not until forty-eight hours later.

During my third round of this heavy dose of antibiotics, upon taking the second pill, twenty-four hours after leaving the pharmacist, I began experiencing 25–30 Temporary Ischemic Attacks (TIAs). Essentially, these were stroke-like symptoms that would happen every time I stood up; they lasted for five to seven seconds each, leaving me unable to walk and extremely dizzy. This scared the heck out of me, way more than having a paralyzed leg. With the paralyzed leg, I knew what was causing it, but with the TIAs, I had no idea why they were happening.

I immediately visited a neurologist, who could not diagnose a reason or solution. The best guess he could come up with was that impulses were being sent through my veins upon standing up. I spoke with other neurologists, who came to the same farfetched conclusion. They prescribed me a statin medication (the kind you take for high cholesterol), in hopes it would relax the constriction of my veins. The statin medication brought down the TIAs from twenty-five to thirty per day to three to five per day, but I concluded any number of strokes, even one a day, was completely unacceptable. There was absolutely no way I was going to live like that.

I was angry and scared, but I was also determined to find a solution to this bizarre problem.

Learning About the Gut

I began to study and educate myself, which led me down many rabbit holes, some being informative, and others not so much. One rabbit hole was about gut microbiota, and I began to study how our brains are fed and how the good bacteria in our bodies outnumber our cells one hundred to one. These good bacteria feed our brains, boost our immune systems, and fight disease, along with many other supporting functions.

Since I spent three months wiping out all the bacteria in my body with antibiotics due to the shin injury, I decided this was the culprit.

I turned myself into a science experiment and focused on replacing all the good bacteria with probiotics along with diet, while also re-establishing the supportive growth medium with prebiotics (prebiotics feed probiotics).

Over the next two months, the TIAs slowly but surely disappeared, an experiment that I was delighted had worked. Then, I promptly wanted to forget these TIAs ever happened. After this experience, I always felt slightly unstable when walking. I chalked it up to my leg injury years before and attempted to ignore it. I kept doing CrossFit, as my motto of "never stop moving" was always there. I remembered the sticker I put on the top tube of my bike during Ironman, which became ingrained in my brain forever:

> "No one cares if you quit,
> but you will always know."

Multiple Sclerosis Diagnosis

In April 2017, two and a half years after the strokes, I visited the neurologist again to have an MRI of my brain completed, just as a checkup. Three days after the MRI, I received the call and heard the nurse tell me she was from the doctor's office. They had my MRI results, and I was not worried. I had received this call before, and it had never gone poorly, just a neutral or benign result, which told me I needed to keep looking. So that day was no different, and I approached the call with neutrality and a laissez-faire attitude. When she told me that the MRI showed signs of MS, I had no idea what that meant. I had only heard of MS on TV, and that was the extent of my understanding. I did not even know what the acronym "MS" stood for or what it meant.

After minimal research, I found out quickly that MS stood for multiple sclerosis. As I looked a little further, I read the definition of multiple sclerosis: a chronic, typically progressive disease involving damage to the sheaths of nerve cells in the brain and spinal cord. It said my body was attacking itself, causing multiple brain lesions or brain scarring.

Angels and teachers were watching over me again in this instance. Two weeks before the MRI, my sister-in-law sent my then-wife and me the book *Medical Medium*, by Anthony William. When asked why she sent the book, she reluctantly admitted that something in her head woke her up in the middle of the night and ordered her to do it.

After catching my breath after being diagnosed with multiple sclerosis, and time had passed, the shock and fear of the diagnosis subsided. Then, my brain kicked back into overdrive, and I began ferociously researching again. William's book was a part of that, and I began to learn about how nutrient-dense, toxin-free food can heal disease, even MS. I studied doctors who had reversed their own diagnosis of MS, to go on and lead seemingly normal lives.

The lesions in my brain were considered severe, and after visiting multiple top MS specialists from California to Colorado, it became obvious that the medical community did not know what was causing it or how to cure it effectively. The prognosis by the medical community was that it was an autoimmune disease, and my immune system was attacking the myelin sheath in my brain and spine.

All of my appointments ended predominantly the same: You have multiple lesions on your brain and spinal cord showing Primary Progressive MS.

The newest, most promising drug was Ocrevus, an immunosuppressant medication. The delivery of the medication was conducted by a 2.5-hour intravenous injection. Once the medication was in a person's body, it suppressed the B-cell of the immune system.

As the doctor explained what this meant and suggested I take the drug, I asked about details. I was then handed the "medication information insert" supplied by the manufacturer. Imagine a sheet of thin paper, folded like a complicated map. This insert explained all the side effects and results from the drug trials and tests for Ocrevus conducted on patients with MS. The drug's information, delivered in small font, showed that patients with Primary Progressive MS experienced only 27 percent effectiveness of the drug halting the disease's progression. In 38 percent of the patients, the drug made them worse, and for everyone else, it did nothing.

I did not find those odds comforting, and I felt shamed and discouraged for not saying "yes" to the drug. I asked the doctor, if she had a 27 percent chance that she would make it safely home, would she leave her office today? Her prognosis for me, if I decided not to take the drug, was not promising, with the chance of being wheelchair-bound by Christmas, which was only seven months away.

Due to the events that happened with the TIAs two and a half years earlier, I began to question my "inevitable" prognosis. I decided to look at reasons and causes other than what the specialists were telling me.

I felt the doctors were asking more questions than providing certainty. So, after much thought and many discussions with my then-wife, I decided to keep looking for a better option. After my first appointment, I had already decided to educate myself as much as possible. What I wanted, and still want, is to be with my grandkids and not be in a wheelchair! (At the time I am writing this, my kids are seventeen and fifteen.)

Soon after being diagnosed, I began to explore what other options there were for MS patients. I treated food as a science experiment and paid close attention to how I felt after eating certain foods. All of these steps were small and intentional, but deep within, I knew I was on the right path for me. I learned how to stop and avoid negative threads of information and how to move toward information that provided results and possibility. I vowed through this journey to never stop moving, so I had to keep trying. Deep down, I *knew* this was right; if you've ever before had that deep feeling of *knowing,* you know what I mean. But there were times I also felt lost, searching for the next step, and my fear left me in a depressed, negative mindset.

I knew this negative state and stress was going to affect my ability to control my diagnosis and feel better. It was not until I came to the conclusion that my feelings and thoughts were 100 percent up to me and no one else. Approaching the situation from my authentic Self allowed me to take a step back and view the encounter from a different, more productive lens. If I approached my interactions with my negative self-perception, I would not have kept moving forward and allowed all hope of overcoming this disease to fade away.

During all these events, it ultimately came down to me and how I viewed them.

I thought about who I was, what I wanted, and what was needed in order for me to achieve my goal of walking, well into my old age. I thought about the choices I was making. I reflected on how my time was spent and what topics and thoughts deserved my attention. As I became clearer on what I wanted, it was easier to know where to spend my time and energy. There was little debate about the logical choices that lay ahead, although at times I was not 100 percent clear on the path, and where it would lead. Every step brought another set of questions, and in some cases, an incredible person to guide me through it.

I began studying and experimenting with food as medicine and paid attention to what I ate and how I felt. For example, if I felt dizzy, tired, angry, depressed, or not myself, I avoided the foods that caused those feelings. I also took a journey within myself and studied Who I Was and What I Wanted. That journey would be the most important and hardest work I have ever done.

> Before taking the time to understand my true Self, I found I was easily swayed by what others said and suggested. My thoughts reinforced these suggestions and my self-acceptance.

I felt like I was being tossed on an ocean, with no sail or rudder to steer. Being out of control left me with depression and anger. I could no longer identify with the athlete that I once was. This lack of a core foundation of Self left me feeling lost, and changing my identity was not on my mind.

Holding on to my past was like tightly holding on to melting ice cream, struggling to keep it together. Everything I tried that was based on my old identity—long training rides, attempting to run again, the Ironman—was a part of my past; I tried to fill a bottomless pit of self-love and acceptance. This struggle of trying to hold on to my past increased my anger and depression. Although the accomplishments felt good at the moment, they did not last, and I wanted more. I did not know Who I Was; I could not answer the next important question: What I Wanted.

Conclusion

Through my early journey, my past became my reason for moving forward. This past was an ever-moving target, because I held on to external accomplishments as my identity. This past identity was filled with great accomplishments, but it was not *me*. It took multiple injuries and the diagnosis of a disease to wake me up to what was important.

The important part of life is not what I accomplished but my own true, authentic Self. All my external accomplishments, although great memories, were easily taken away in a matter of seconds, leaving me feeling lost.

> Where in your own life have you
> held on to something as your truth and
> sense of Self, to watch it fade away?

When we hold on to something outside ourselves and use it as an anchor of Who We Are, it is similar to building a house on sand. It takes one event before your house eventually crumbles, and then what are you left with? We rely on our passions, love, and priorities to be external objects, as we forget about loving ourselves. By looking within, anchoring our identity to Who We Are and our true sense of Self, we develop a foundation that cannot be shaken.

As we look within, we begin to realize that the only way out is through the discovery of Self. This discovery of Self involves self-love, compassion, joy, and a realization that you have a higher Self. As we let go of and surrender to this higher Self, we begin to understand the most important part of anyone's life is themselves.

> The *You* that you are when you have
> a love for Self that leaves you in
> awe can never be taken away.

This foundation allows you to see the next step, and then another, on your journey of building the Belief and knowledge you need to overcome the most difficult challenges you may be facing.

All of our challenges are real and not to be ignored, but our perception of these challenges leaves us feeling like a victim—that the event is happening *to* you and not *for* you.

Through my journey, one of the best discoveries was the realization that all my injuries, setbacks, and eventually, the disease, was happening *for* me. This realization had me walk the path of discovering Self, which sometimes was seen more fully by sitting quietly. I had to learn to ask myself difficult questions, while allowing myself patience, compassion, and love, as I walked through the storm. I realized this path was not linear, sometimes with three steps forward then two and one half back, with turns that came abruptly, and moments of being lost. Every one of these struggles was building a foundation of self-love, joy, and compassion. During these steps, I found faith in Self—a realization that there was a higher Self, and love was the only true answer.

I decided to go into the storm of Life. What I found as I walked that path was a Belief and knowledge that I would be okay, and that I am worth every second and moment. My journey has left me in tears, swirling in deep emotions I surrendered to, accepting what was to come. As my belief grew, so did my trust in myself, which had me listening more than talking, loving more than judging, and exhibiting a compassion that left me in awe.

As we walk this road together, we are going to discover ourselves. During this journey, we may invoke deep-seated emotions, and during this time, compassion and love for Self is the answer to get through them. This choice is not an easy one, but it will be the most important one you take.

You are not alone,
and I am proud you are
choosing to take this journey.

Chapter 2

Becoming Aware

"Be grateful for whoever comes,
because each has been sent as a guide from beyond."

– Mawlana Jalal-al-Din Rumi, *"The Guest House"*

"Fear keeps us focused on the past or worried
about the future. If we can acknowledge our fear,
we can realize that right now we are okay. Right now,
today, we are still alive, and our bodies are working
marvelously. Our eyes can still see the beautiful sky.
Our ears can still hear the voices of our loved ones."

~Thich Nhat Hanh, Fear: Essential Wisdom for Getting Through the Storm

Awareness is a Choice

We all have choices, every minute of every day. We choose what we think, how we are being, and how we view healing or recovering from a disease or medical issue. At the beginning of my multiple sclerosis diagnosis, it felt as if I was given a sentence by a judge. The idea that I had a choice in any part of my life during that time seemed like a ridiculous thought. Having a positive mindset and a choice that leads to possibility is difficult, when you are reminded regularly about why you are afraid.

Also, the fear that is indirectly imposed upon you as a patient becomes further ingrained and reinforced when you do not view yourself as someone who can do anything about it. It was as if I was leaving my life and desires to fate and doctors I trusted. Sometimes, we feel like we are being pulled in the direction of our negative thoughts, and the worry of our next doctor's appointment can leave us feeling lonelier and more hopeless.

> Over time, I realized that a positive feeling and a belief that I could do something about what I was experiencing started with me, my beliefs and identity of who I thought I was. My self-imposed identity led to my thoughts and the desire to take a small step, or not.

The identity of Who We Think We Are can drive what we think, which can lead to how we behave, and our behaviors lead to our actions and results. When we are in the middle of the storm, we do not see our thoughts and identities affecting our decisions. We become mad with justification, proving to ourselves why life is complicated and a fight.

What makes this journey more complicated is when our health is not where we want it to be, and we rely on others to label the diagnoses, give us the "magic pill," or tell us how we are supposed to feel.

A few years before the diagnosis of multiple sclerosis, I was hiking a difficult trail in Colorado, and I came upon an older gentleman hiking down the trail. He was doing well, with a huge smile. We began talking and after a few minutes, I asked him how old he was. He said, "Eighty-four."

When I asked him his secret, he looked at me proudly, and said, "Always do." Then, he proudly told me he does this hike every day.

What did he tell himself when he woke up? Was it possible for him, or did he view it as a negative chore? This man's thoughts about who he was drove him to live in *possibility*.

> Once we come to the realization that we have a choice, where do we begin the journey of feeling better, like we remember or desire ourselves to feel?

The first step in the journey of controlling a disease is the awareness of where you are, both mentally and physically. Once we are aware of where we are, we then have a choice of how we want to be. We can see the first step, no matter how small it is. So many times, we want to go from *the state we are in* to *completely healed* in one leap. But by trying to take this large leap, we do not see the journey or steps it will take to discover the root cause of the disease. During this leap, we ignore the lessons the disease tries to show us.

By burying our heads in the sand, hiding from fear, pain, and anger, a disease can stop us from seeing the most important part: *ourselves*. By slowing down, we allow the teachers, mentors, and guides to come into our lives, and we accept their guidance, or at least, we can be led to this important first step.

What Is Awareness?

The Merriam-Webster Dictionary defines awareness as "knowledge and understanding that something is happening or exists."

When we know something is happening, then we can make a choice of how we want to be. No one tells us how we are *supposed* to think or act. We make the choice to be a certain way, based on what is happening in our external environment.

When we feel our choice is taken away from us, we experience stress and a lack of alignment, which we will be discussing in later chapters.

Where Does Awareness Begin?

When we become aware that we have a choice, we can choose to walk or not to walk a path of discovery and finding ourselves. As the great Buddha once said, "By oneself is evil done; by oneself is one defiled. By oneself is evil left undone; by oneself is one made pure. Purity and impurity depend on oneself; no one can purify another" (as translated in Access to Insight, 1996).

The story of the hiker illustrates this point. He made a decision of how he wanted to be at eighty-four years old. This Awareness—of what he wanted in his life and who he identified himself as being—drove him to who he was and the actions he took, every day.

He could have very easily woken up that morning, with every pain and reason not to go hike, but he didn't. He continued on the path that he wanted for himself.

Just like you. *You* have a choice. You have a choice in where you want to be and who you want to be as an individual. No one in this beautiful universe has the right to dictate Who You Are; this is your own soul's purpose.

> Yes, your diagnosis is very real,
> and your pains are very real. But each of us
> has the choice whether or not we are defined
> by them, and whether or not they shape our
> existence in Who We Are as an individual,

After healing my paralyzed leg, experiencing TIAs that paralyzed the right side of my body, and then the diagnosis of MS, as mentioned in Chapter 1, I had every reason to be afraid.

And I was.

I was too young to allow the fear to shape my existence into who I thought I was. This fear was real; this fear was debilitating; this fear, at times, left me frozen, worrying about a future that had not happened yet.

At this time, I had made a decision not to be defined or live the rest of my life this way. So, I began exploring why, the root cause, for everything that was happening. My Awareness of what was happening to me drove me to a first step, then another. These steps began to craft my reality, unintentionally. Who I thought I was, the steps I took, always led me to another step. As the wonderful quote, often attributed to Dr. Martin Luther King Jr., says: "We do not need to see the entire staircase, just the first step."

Although at the time, I was feeling alone, frustrated, and angry about what was happening to me. Yet, I still continued to take a step. Sometimes these steps were small and presented in a very gentle way, and sometimes these steps were big, but each step led me to a new discovery of not only who I was as an individual, but also, they led me along a path of discovering how to feel better and overcome my symptoms.

As you will read in a later chapter, this discovery led me to a better understanding of bacteria inside our bodies that promotes neurological health, food as medicine, meditation, healing energies, and also, another self-discovery that was the greatest and most beautiful lesson I could have learned.

The Debilitating Effects of Fear

What helped during this time of Awareness was knowing that I was not alone, as I began experiencing bouts of sadness, anger, and depression. My temper and patience shortened because I worried about what was wrong with me. As my frustration grew, I was not patient or nice, as I expressed these feelings of frustrations to my family. I also noticed the other factors that played a part in both my physical and mental well-being. For example, during the period of my life with the TIAs, if I ate gluten (pizza, bread, beer, etc.), I would feel a slight case of vertigo but not a full-blown TIA episode, and the frustration and sadness became more intense.

I was scared, even though if you would have asked me at the time, I would have said, "No, I am fine." I wanted to hide my self-perceived weakness from everyone, including myself. I did not want to come to the realization that this may be the rest of my life. I ignored and disregarded the love that my family poured on me. All I could think about was a future that I had no control over. The only thing I could control was my outward appearance and what others thought of me. So, I bolted on my mask and pretended to be what I thought others wanted.

During these months, while I experienced the TIAs, I tried—on the outside—to portray the confident young executive I pretended to be. On the inside, I was depressed, frustrated, and felt that I was not enough. I felt broken and lonely. I desperately wanted life to rewind itself to the time before all this started. The fear of the future and the regret from the past started to lead me toward a hopeless victim mindset.

I did not know what to do or where to begin. I had a far-fetched idea that the extreme amount of antibiotics that was being given to me at the time could be one place to start. I knew that within twelve hours of taking a heavy dose of antibiotics, the TIAs started. This was all I had to go on, but it was a place to start looking. This self-prescribed cause, and my reasons were not agreed upon by neurologists, but what was my risk in continuing to look at this possible cause?

When my first appointment finally happened with the neurologist regarding the TIAs, the neurologist had no idea what was happening, and a statin drug was suggested. I was looking for a magic pill, and there was no hesitation; I agreed to start the medication. I did not hesitate, because I was afraid, and I reached for anything that might help my situation. When I asked the doctor about the causation between the antibiotics and the TIAs, I was dismissed and told that antibiotics do not cause neurological issues or TIAs.

When we bury our head or hide from disease or ailment, our symptoms may become more prevalent, as if the disease is trying to grab our attention. It is only the act of facing this fear that allows us to begin to understand where the root of the fear lies, where our fear comes from. By slowing down and looking inside ourselves, we may be led to a book, online article, or some person who has overcome our specific ailment.

There have been many times I have read a book or article, not fully comprehending the depth of wisdom or knowledge it was attempting to bestow upon me, but that book or article led me to another step. My Awareness led me to important lessons, including the ability to listen to what I was told or understand what I was reading.

As you begin your journey toward Self-Awareness or deeper awareness of any ailment, be patient with yourself. Look beyond. It may take multiple times reading or listening to this wisdom over many months.

If you feel you missed a key element, or for some reason, you feel drawn back to a specific topic, publication, or way to obtain knowledge, I challenge you to go back and try to see it from a new angle. As we are on the path, we are growing and changing to be the person we are, and that involves becoming wiser from within. I remember many times reading something again during my journey of self-discovery and finding other lessons within that I was not able to hear before. If I had stopped looking, some important lessons could have been missed.

Medications & Gut Health

When I was experiencing the TIAs, I was not receiving the answer I desired, or at least, an answer I felt good about, from the neurologists. So, I began studying about Keflex—the antibiotic I was given. Had Keflex caused this TIA response in anyone else? There were loose threads, and my research kept taking me back to bacteria. I followed the thread of bacteria, since antibiotics kill bacteria, both good and bad.

I needed more of a reason, just in case the re-establishment of my gut microbiome did not work like I was hypothesizing. I began to assess how I got there and what other factors may have contributed to the TIAs, along with the antibiotics. As I reestablished my good bacteria, I also began reading books regarding stress and mental health, such as *The Presence Process* by Michael Brown, *The Surrender Experiment* and *Untethered Soul* by Michael A. Singer, along with teachings by Buddha on Self and meditation, and philosopher Ding Ming-Dao on the essence of Taoism. At the time I did not realize it, but I began a journey of self-discovery that took many abrupt turns, derailments, and an Awareness of my feelings and emotions that I was not used to addressing.

As I read books on stress, shame, loneliness, fear, and the damaging effects these have on the body—books like those from Dr. Brené Brown, Dr. Joe Dispenza, and Louise Hay—I realized I had all these feelings and bodily damage. At this time, I rated my feelings in all of these areas as *high* or *extreme*.

According to Bruce McEwen, a neuroscientist from Rockefeller University:

> *"Because stress changes the way the brain's neurons communicate with each other, chronic stress can cause our brains, nervous systems, and our behavior to adjust to a vigilant and reactive state" (as cited in Caldwell, 2018).*

This constant vigilance can lead to devastating mental and physical health conditions for the person experiencing it. As I researched further, I found that when stress becomes chronic, a person's fight-or-flight system is amped up all the time. The same hormones that are so important for the fight-or-flight response can lead to digestive issues, trouble sleeping, and a weakened immune system, making a person more susceptible to viruses like the flu and other chronic health problems.

Stress & Its Impacts

At this time, I had been experiencing a high level of stress for as long as I could remember, along with feeling isolated and alone. There was no one to talk to about what I was experiencing and the fear I had. I did not know how to talk about what was going on with me mentally, and my family was becoming frustrated because they could not or did not know how to help me. I was being led toward a therapist, but because of stigma I had internalized around needing a therapist, because of my upbringing, I never gave the option a chance or searched for someone I could talk to about how I was feeling.

Due to my low sense of self-worth, I could not handle the thought of needing a therapist. So, I kept researching mental health. I studied about people's need for connection and acceptance, living in the Present Moment, meditation, and ways to reduce my stress, in hopes that I could find an answer on my own. My research did provide some relief and understanding, but I was covering and numbing the real reason. I thought that if I could gain control again, my life would go back to the way it was. Wow, was I naïve. I was still masking the real reasons.

The areas I tried to control and address included stress, my young kids—who were eight and ten at the time—what I ate, the fear and stress of living paycheck to paycheck, my relationship with my then-wife, and my anger, depression, and outward appearance. I was in denial about my anxiety and fears that something was wrong with me. The thoughts of living this way for the rest of my life were buried deep, masked over, and avoided.

I did not abandon Western medicine, as my experiment on gut microbiome had very little risk and a far-stretching theory.

As I continued my gut microbiome experiment over the next couple months, I found myself having fewer TIA episodes, and my need for taking the statin medication was decreasing. I was excited because I felt that I was onto something. My mind was rarely at rest, and I had to give my brain a job to avoid the downward spiral of self-deprecating thoughts and depression. As I continued with my experiment, I noticed the TIAs go away over the next thirty days, and I stopped taking the statin medication. I was also motivated to stop taking the medication after researching the negative long-term side effects from the statin drug.

Just because the TIAs ended did not mean I was done researching meditation and my mental health. I had awakened a sleeping dragon that would not let me ignore how I felt any longer. No matter how large or thick my mask was, it did not cover up what I was feeling, and I could not hide from those feelings.

> Often during our Awareness,
> we are led down subsequent paths that catch our
> attention. Through your own discovery

of seeking the root cause, I encourage you to
explore these paths, while staying focused
on what you are seeking to find.

If I wanted to get a handle on my stress, I felt I needed to increase my sense of self-worth. I have no idea why I began leaning this way, but I started to think and make a list of what I knew to be true about me and who I thought I was, or in the least, who I aspired to be. Some areas were obvious—like being a loving, kind, and a joyful father and husband—but other areas involved my Ego, like being a driven athlete and entrepreneur.

I could not stop the constant mental chatter that reminded me of the areas where I failed or made mistakes. It was a challenge to keep the negative thoughts of bankrupting a company from overtaking the good I had done with overcoming the TIAs. By becoming aware of what was the root cause of the TIAs, I continued my journey of my mental health that I desperately needed. The constant, limiting thoughts were frustrating and added to the stress and my fear, leaving me feeling that I was not enough or good enough.

It was easy to think about all the times I made a mistake and felt I screwed up, and I knew this thought process was not helping me. I wanted to find a way to address these negative thoughts. Ignoring them, masking them, or telling them to stop was not enough, and at times, impossible. The fear that I felt was out of control. I was hiding the fear, and I thought I had few choices. All that I had was my family, who were supportive, but what was happening to me was hard to explain, which added frustration to my fear.

At times, I felt alone, and the more I heard the doctor's uncertainty, it only deepened this feeling of being alone and afraid.

I knew I had to make a choice, either remain a victim or get to work and deal with the awful feeling I was slipping into. At times, I felt like a boat on the ocean with no sail or rudder to steer my direction. Little did I know that the research I was conducting was about the outside world and my response to it, when this was only a small part of what I would discover I needed.

This choice started with research and looking for books and teachers that may have an answer. The books, friends, and unexpected teachers led me to the constant negative mental chatter, which I knew was not helping me, and this awareness of the negative internal chatter and damaging effects led me to start making a different choice. I started thinking about what I wanted in my life, not just from an external desire, house, car, etc., but also, what I wanted for myself and my family. I wanted to be happy and respected and to have joy in my life. I wanted to hike and run with my grandkids, and due to the TIAs, I thought all this was in jeopardy of never happening.

> I realized my fear kept me from seeing any sort of possibility, and I thought more about what I could not do and what I was losing, instead of all the good I had in my life.

The Self & Changing the Self

Around the age of eight to twelve, individuals begin to develop the foundation of our perception of Who We Think We Are, our perceived core identity, our self-schema. *Self-schema* is a psychology term, which interacts with self-esteem, self-knowledge, and the social self to form the *Self* as a whole. It includes the past, present, and future selves, where future selves (or possible selves) represent an individual's ideas of who they might become, what they would like to become, or what they are afraid of becoming.

The concept of *Self* was first introduced to Western society by psychologists Carl Rogers and Abraham Maslow. Carl Rogers (1995) wrote, "The curious paradox is that when I accept myself just as I am, then I can change." These gentlemen had significant influence in popularizing the idea of self-concept in the West.

One thing that the research never tells us is how long we need to hold on to an identity that is not serving us.

As I look back, I can see where my way of thinking became misguided. I recently looked at a picture of myself smiling and confident when I was eight, and I began to wonder what I was thinking and the freedom I had allowed myself to act and be. Subconsciously, I desired to be that little boy again. I needed to go back to the beginning and address these feelings, one by one.

I was probably living in the moment and not worried about what others thought or the failures I experienced. I lived without concern about my impression on others, enjoying everything I did right. I am sure there were moments when I became upset, frustrated, sad, and hurt, but they were just that—moments. I did not hold on to these negative thoughts. I let them pass, some slowly, and some in an instant. I understand that I was only eight, with no pressures of family, money, job, or security. I also lived a privileged life, not worried about abuse, hunger, and pain, which at times, sadly, cannot be avoided.

I realize now that all these thoughts and constant questions are because of me. My reactions and thoughts to events happening, self-imposed labels and stories I told myself were the driving forces of my fear. All of these are my perception of the situation. If you were there with me, documenting my entire life story from birth (really creepy), your story would be different from mine.

So, why can't we make a new story, now?

> I am not suggesting we forget the past
> or the memories we hold dear to our hearts.
> I am suggesting we do not allow our past
> to hold us hostage anymore.

One Change at a Time

For a possible first step, a suggestion given by Steve Chandler, a prominent thought leader, modern-day philosopher, teacher, and author recommends his readers to: "Write down ten things you would do in your life if you had no fear. Then pick one of them and do it."

The past is just a position to learn from, to help you avoid strife and pain or bring more joy and laughter. Why are we holding on so tightly to our past and the identities we crafted when we were children? It would be like going to my daughter's middle school and asking ten-year-old and twelve-year-old children to plan my next year, based on who they think I am. That would be asinine! But, we do it every day.

Have you ever looked in the mirror and called yourself by the nickname you may have gained or given yourself in middle school? I know some individuals who still hold on to their nicknames, identifying themselves to that name.

My self-imposed identity was mine, and I created it. I was not approached by my teachers, bullies, the popular kids, or family telling me who I was supposed to be.

When I looked back, no one cared, and if I approached them today, they would not remember the situation or story that I labeled myself with. The labels and fear that we self-impose are just that: labels. When we grow up, we become comfortable with labels, and at times, rely upon them. The categorizations of "who we think we are" or "how we are supposed to act" become the norms and standards. *I am an introvert; I am not detail oriented; I talk a lot; I am not...* Fill in the blank. These are labels that we adopted ourselves, and no one told us to be that way.

> We assign labels to our fears, and we become good at avoiding this feeling of fear. Our fears are not something to avoid, but fear is an emotion that can be used as a guidepost for areas to pay attention to.

This positive choice did not change my carefully poised facade that nothing was wrong. It was the first time I was truly scared, and I felt my grip tighten on controlling all I could.

I became utterly focused on hiding behind my "mask," making decisions about my life based on what others would think. I justified my way of thinking, which reinforced my lack of self-worth and the negative thoughts that plagued me during this time. I thought pleasing others was serving me and helping me attain the life I did not have, but that I desperately wanted. Every time a normal, everyday obstacle presented itself, I blamed both myself and others, holding on to my victim mentality and my scarcity mindset. I became excellent at hiding behind this "mask" of mine. I could not understand why I was very successful on paper, but still living paycheck to paycheck.

> I was desperately seeking happiness, acceptance, credibility, wealth, respect, while wearing a blindfold. This way of hiding, ironically, brought me greater stress than if I had just owned who I was.

How Diagnosis Forces/Rushes Change

The opposite can happen when someone is diagnosed with a disease. Your doctor may seem like the kids on the playground; he or she makes a statement that leaves you feeling a certain way, mentally. This feeling or imposed label starts to create your list of choices. These choices become limited by the additional labels or identity we are inflicting upon ourselves.

> What if we believed we were the cause of everything in our lives? There is no right or wrong. There's no judgment. It just *is*.

If you are the cause, then you have control, and you can cause anything you want in your life to begin happening, based on your choices. Those who think, "This is happening *to* me" can be left feeling and thinking they have no control.

Those who think, "This is happening *for* me" remain in control and begin thinking about ways to change their situation.

> No matter the diagnosis, we have a choice of
> how we want to live our lives *right now.*

This is a difficult concept to wrap your mind around, but think of it this way: If I come downstairs tomorrow morning at 7 a.m., and I scream at the top of my lungs, I am the cause of the incident, and the outcome will be a discussion with my family—one that will not turn out in my favor.

On the other side of the spectrum, if I come downstairs tomorrow morning at 7 a.m., and I kiss my kids and make a cup of coffee for my partner, then deliver it with a kiss, I will still be the cause, but the outcome will be her appreciation and love.

Which outcome would you rather have? I know what my choice is.

You can give me every excuse in the book, every reason and all of them are justified, and for some, you may feel it is impossible because of how you feel. Have you asked yourself, who is the one letting this label affect their lives and possibly their fear of the situation?

> Who has to wake up every morning
> and handle the diagnosis? You.

Chapter 2 Exercise

List of Past Events, Divided

The first step toward taking control of yourself and the situation is becoming aware of how you may have gotten here. Start by getting a journal—any notebook you like will do, but it should be a specific notebook only you use.

This first exercise asks you to take the time now in your journal to make a list.

On a new page or blank piece of paper, draw a line down the center of the page to divide it into two areas for separate lists. On the left side, you'll make a list of negative situations that led you to this point, and on the right side, you'll make a list of positive situations that led you to this point.

If your situations are only negative, that is okay. You are now aware of them, and they can no longer hide. You have a choice about how you want these situations to affect you. If stress is so damaging to our bodies, minds, and souls, we cannot begin to change our stressors or address them, until we know what they are.

As you make your list, think back to moments when you were young, perhaps between the ages of five and fourteen. Some events may have happened earlier or later, and if they were negative, it could lead to subconscious trauma and reactions. In cases of abuse or other traumatic events, they could be difficult to write down. Take your time with these sensitive areas. Offer compassion to yourself. This list is for *you*, and no one has to see it.

If the list you create stirs up difficult memories that you want to bury deep, become aware of the moments you are trying to hide. These moments can be roots of areas to address with a therapist or coach.

Feel where these moments are located within your body. Do you feel tightening in your stomach, below your rib cage, in your throat, or near your heart? Note your physical reactions.

These areas may bring up difficult moments you no longer wish to address, but if you do not deal with these areas, they could continue affecting you. For example, when I was young, my perception was that I was not loved, and I felt abandoned when I needed love. I felt it in my body, in my solar plexus—the space right below my ribs—where our self-worth resides. As I grew, I sought approval from anyone; I wanted to be accepted. This led me to act out in specific ways, to gain this acceptance, instead of just being my true, authentic Self.

Conclusion: Your Gift

We are going to explore these areas and develop a reason to think differently about your situation. We are going to explore what gets in our way from being the person we so desperately want to be. Our exploration will take us to questions that we have avoided and beliefs that no longer serve us. We are going to look at the masks we bolt on and the stresses we live with.

You have a gift, a reason for being here, your love to share, and the hope you give others. No matter your situation or diagnosis, we all have an opportunity to learn from what is happening to us and inspire others by how we live in these moments.

It is the smile we give when our hearts open to love. Not because we think it is the right thing to do, but because we want to. If what I just said brings doubt, scrutiny, or the belief that this is impossible, that is okay. Through all the moments of our lives, we can only share love if we first begin to love ourselves. As we explore how we can change our beliefs, identity, and mindset of our situations, we will be exploring ourselves first and how we love ourselves.

As we take this journey, I would like you to remember the humorous advice, "Those that matter don't mind, and those that mind, don't matter."

So, dance in public, smile at those you pass. Sing and laugh as often as you can. This is your life, and I want you to live it fully until the end.

Chapter 3

Letting Go

"What's the greater risk? Letting go of what people think—or letting go of how I feel, what I believe, and who I am?"

– Dr. Brené Brown, *The Gifts of Imperfection*

Hanging on too Tight

My friend tells a beautiful story of horseback riding for the first time. She was terrified of horses but was determined to overcome this fear. After addressing the fear, she found a ranch in Montana that offered horseback riding. As she swung her leg up onto the horse, the fear caused her to squeeze her legs on each side of the horse and hold the reins tightly. Those who are familiar with horse riding know this signals the horse to run. As the horse took off, she remembers hearing the instructor urging her to let go. At this point, the horse was in a run, headed for a fence. My friend had a choice to either let go or be seriously injured.

Her first thought was, "No way in hell am I letting go," but as she rapidly approached the fence, she began to loosen the grip of her legs on the horse, slowing the animal down, and eventually relaxing her legs completely, which signaled the horse to walk.

This story is an excellent example of circumstances in life where we tighten our grip in an effort to maintain control. This grip we maintain keeps us focused on the specific moment we are holding on to, not allowing us to see other possibilities. This short-sighted focus may let opportunities for laughter, healing, love, and anything else we are searching for, slide past our Awareness. When we squeeze tight in fear, we stop listening to ourselves, our intuition, and possibly our families, friends, doctors, and anyone else who is trying to help us.

I have noticed these moments in my own life, and at times, feel as if I am gripping tightly to the reins of the horse as it races forward. My tight grip has me running past the moments to enjoy more of my life. I don't stop to look at the beautiful planet we live on, the smile on a child's face, the beauty of silence, and the warmth that comes from loving myself.

If I feel pain in my legs or a lack of balance or light-headed from doing too much, I grip tighter to the reality of what I am feeling. This tighter grip leads me to fear that this might be the way it is, and I stop looking at why this may be happening. My fear leads me to stress and negative thoughts I tell myself. This stress leads me to inflammation, and the cycle continues. When we take a step back and look at these moments—no matter how bad they are—as opportunities, guideposts, and reasons to slow down and take a breath—we allow this opportunity to provide us a lesson. If we continue to ignore how we currently feel—either good or bad—we allow this opportunity to slip away, as we grip tighter.

We do not give ourselves these opportune moments to enjoy life. We do not slow down enough to understand what may have happened that caused our joy or pain.

> Where might you be holding on so tightly
> that everything seems impossible, all the while,
> moving faster and faster toward a fence?

My Healing Journey Continued

When I left the neurologist's office after the discussion about my TIAs, I knew I had a choice: Stay on the statin medication indefinitely with no answers or begin looking into other options and the risks. If the doctors were at a loss, and I had no specific direction to follow, I had to begin looking for a possible cause.

The best way to describe my journey of finding an answer is that it was like looking for an answer in a book, in the largest library you have ever seen, with no reference section. The perception of my past began to filter my experiences, either perpetuating or deflating the opportunities I thought I had available to me. This feeling the doctors left me with—feelings of scarcity and limited perceived options—was crafting my reality, and I could either allow this past to dictate my world or not. The persona I developed based on others' opinions kept me from being curious and open. Then, this lack of curiosity and feeling that I was smart enough kept me from getting out of my own way in order to heal and live the life I desired. I was driving my choices out of the fear that feeling "this way" could be the rest of my life. I kept gripping tighter to the horse, as it ran out of control.

How did this negative aspect affect my ability to move forward and see the possibility that I *was* smart enough to take my life into my own hands?

If you do not address this negative aspect of yourself, it may cause chronic problems that affect you for a lifetime.

Many thought leaders like Buddha and Jesus, as well as prominent yogis, describe wisdom as being based in *Awareness*. They prescribe slowing down, meditating, praying, and gratitude, in every situation. It was said by the Buddha, "To enjoy good health, to bring true happiness to one's family, to bring peace to all, one must first discipline and control one's own mind. If a man can control his mind, he can find the way to enlightenment, and all wisdom and virtue will naturally come to him" (as cited in Kyōkai, 2005).

I was allowing the natural ebb and flow of life to drag me down, and I was left feeling inferior. This feeling of inadequacy was leading me down a dangerous road. The difficult moment of experiencing the TIAs left me feeling out of control, depressed, angry, and lost. As I studied further, I realized I was letting these negative thoughts and feelings control me. I stopped, or at least ignored, the teachers who were trying to help me and the thoughts or ideas being presented to me. I was driving my car using the rearview mirror.

When in your life have you looked for an item, with feverish desire, only to find it when you were not looking for it? My kids are great at pointing out that the sunglasses I have been looking for are sitting on top of my head.

Getting Out of My Own Way

During my research, I came across business, religious, and spiritual leaders who used a positive mindset and gratitude to overcome these difficult moments. But was this the answer? All I had to do to overcome my fear was to "think good thoughts" and "be my authentic self"?

I tried to adopt these ways, with little to no success, due to more than thirty-five years of embedded negative thoughts. Although I kept looking for peace and a sense of calm, all I found was more frustration. I was getting stressed about not being stressed out.

How could I surrender enough to get out of my own way? My act of holding on too tight mixed with the negative thoughts that I was "not good enough" or "not smart enough" to find a way to heal, kept me from healing. I was no different than what was going on in the story at the beginning of the chapter. I did not want to let go; I wanted to hold on to my old way of thinking, because it felt *safe*. I had a fear of letting go of the reins and releasing the death grip I had on my life.

I noticed that when I was happy, grateful, and optimistic, beneficial opportunities naturally presented themselves, which at the time, I took for granted. Because I viewed these events as *lucky*, gratitude did not follow.

My desire of not wanting to change became a vicious spiral, leaving me with a victim mentality. As the TIAs continued, I realized my mindset was causing my unfavorable behaviors. The yoyo-ing of my thoughts either resulted in stress or happiness. When the thoughts were negative, this mindset resulted in a cascade of negative behaviors, actions, and outcomes. This led to me feeling lost, with ongoing, perpetuated stress, while I continued to search for an answer.

According to a 2012 study conducted and funded by The National Center for Complementary and Alternative Medicine; National Institute of Mental Health; National Heart, Lung, and Blood Institute; and the MacArthur

Foundation Research Network on Socioeconomic Status and Health, a research team led by Dr. Sheldon Cohen at Carnegie Mellon University found that chronic psychological stress is associated with the body losing its ability to regulate the inflammatory response.

> *"The immune system's ability to regulate inflammation predicts who will develop a cold, but more importantly it provides an explanation of how stress can promote disease," Cohen said. "When under stress, cells of the immune system are unable to respond to hormonal control, and consequently, produce levels of inflammation that promote disease. Because inflammation plays a role in many diseases such as cardiovascular, asthma and autoimmune disorders, this model suggests why stress impacts them as well" (as cited in Carnegie Mellon University, 2012).*

Was I discovering something? Although all the signs pointed to perpetuated unmitigated stress, was I somehow making my situation harder?

Mindset Changes/Negative Thoughts

When my thoughts were negative, I felt tired, unmotivated, not good enough or smart enough. These negative thoughts become habitual when not addressed. As stated in Chapter 2—when I became aware of the root cause of these negative thoughts, I could then begin taking steps to address them, stop the habitual negative cycle, and let go.

If negative thoughts that led to stress were the cause, as my wisdom teachers suggested, could I begin to change my mindset? If I then changed my mindset, what effect would this have? Could I heal a disease instead of causing one?

Dr. Robert H. Shmerling (2020) reported on study in Harvard Health Publishing, which found that stress may cause autoimmune disease, such as lupus or rheumatoid arthritis. The study found a higher incidence of autoimmune diseases among those previously diagnosed with stress-related disorders. At this time, I had not been diagnosed with an autoimmune disease, but the link between stress and disease caught my attention.

If I was feeling stressed out, could the resulting inflammation make my situation with the TIAs more prominent?

To put this study into context, think about a car you want or someone you have not spoken to in a while. When you begin thinking of them or the item desired, you tend to see the car everywhere, or that person calls you out of the blue. So, if the stress and negative thoughts kept making me aware of more negative situations, was my stress perpetuating more stress?

I started to pay attention to my negative thoughts. I became aware of when these thoughts arose and the triggers that caused them. Shaping our thoughts may sound simple, but it is difficult to put into daily practice. I had practiced these negative thoughts for over thirty-five years, and these negative thoughts were always easier to fall into subconsciously.

The positive thoughts I desired took effort, as I practiced them over and over. Like an athlete or musician who wants to achieve mastery, I had to practice the positive aspect of my thoughts. Once we are aware of the triggers that cause the negative thought, then we can see them coming, or at least, identify them when they arise. This level of Awareness is important as we practice this new way of being.

The stress you're experiencing now is based on past experiences, scripts, and fear of possible negative outcomes—not the Present Moment. Perhaps our stress affects our behavior and actions. Your body language may show your stress outwardly, causing you to cross your arms or respond defensively. Entering situations with anxiety from past experience or concern about the future keeps us from experiencing the Present Moment. When we are fully in the present moment, our behaviors and actions reflect curiosity and tranquility. In the Present Moment, you may approach the situation with curiosity and a desire to understand, instead of jumping to conclusions that are often incorrect. During Present-Moment Awareness, we offer compassion and forgiveness to ourselves during these moments.

Belief to Heal

How often do we listen to negative voices in our heads?

The fifteenth-century philosopher René Descartes keenly discussed this issue. Approaching any diagnosis or healing begins with listening, being aware, and looking at a diagnosis from multiple angles. This broad, open view of thinking about your own healing requires you to be curious, while letting go.

Having the stress of the past or the anxiety of the future can affect our behaviors and actions every hour of every day. Do you allow your self-limiting beliefs to stifle your curiosity? Negative thinking and fear can cut off our ability to see all available options. This is particularly true when you have been hit with an unexpected and unwanted diagnosis of a disease. However, your interpretation of the diagnosis and result prescribed to you by the physicians is *your choice*.

I could have stopped looking for an answer or correlation and waited on the doctors. If you are fortunate, your diagnosis has a detailed explanation of what it is and why it happens, along with a treatment to accompany it, but oftentimes, the disease is unexplained. In my case, it was unexplained, and doctors and research were still guessing on the treatment.

If a diagnosis or symptoms leave us feeling scared, like they did for me, we may remain frozen in place and not look for alternatives. What happens if we try something new and fail? But what if this failure is necessary to our survival and well-being? How do we change our mindset to view these self-perceived failures as opportunities to learn?

The challenge comes when we stop learning from failure and hold on tighter. We do not get out of our own way to look at challenges from all angles.

Staying in the Present Moment

I became very fearful when I began thinking about the future or the limited possibilities I had. Fear is like an annoying voice that blocks all logic and thought. Although very real, fear kept *curiosity* and *choice* from existing. When I stepped in the fear of the future, I was unable to step away from the noise and be open to other possibilities. I was limiting my ability to heal, and it had nothing to do with the doctors I met but had everything to do with me. I was the limiting factor. By not mentally or physically being able to get out of my own way, or letting go, I was left feeling angry, sad, and hopeless.

> Effective release happens by living in the Present Moment—not the past or the future. Living in the moment forces us to let go because the moment changes constantly.

Armed with this realization, I thought back to times when I was able to remain in the Present Moment. As I searched personal memories and examples of living in the Present Moment in my life, my thoughts turned to my children. They are my greatest teachers, showing me life in the Present Moment.

When my daughter was seven and my son was ten, my then-wife and I took the kids to Guatemala on a mission trip. During this trip, my daughter made a swing out of a rope at the entrance to the village, along with her new friends—two young girls her age who lived in the town. My daughter did not speak Spanish, and her two new friends did not speak English. It was obvious that there was no concern of the swing not working, just the joy of trying and playing. As they solved the problem of making the swing, they laughed and enjoyed the challenge.

Did it work perfectly on the first try? No! However, they never gave up and paid no mind if anyone noticed their struggles. They did not care what others thought. What they cared about was enjoying each other, solving the problem, and playing on their new invention. Think of what they could have said to themselves:

What if the swing did not work? We cannot communicate. I have never made a swing out of rope. I am not handy or creative. What if I fall and get hurt? What if I look like a fool? What if I fail? I am only seven.

Instead, they approached the task with gusto, and they focused on having fun, being in the present moment. This led to laughing, playing, a sense of accomplishment, and profound joy.

Taking Charge/Making Choices/Curiosity

> Your past either limits your choices or has you looking under every rock. As seen in the story above, choosing to let go is a conscious action.

When we decide to question our doctors and take our health into our own hands, we become open to options and curious about other ways to heal, which allows us to see healing from multiple angles.

We begin looking at possibilities, and our mindset begins to shift. With this shifting mindset, we may be open to reading a few books or researching other healing modalities, trying something that we have never experienced or thought of before.

During this time, be careful using absolute words like "never," "always," or "can't," because these set the stage for our perceived available options. If you were just diagnosed with multiple sclerosis (MS), would it not be beneficial to allow yourself to explore all angles of healing? If you remain curious, you will discover stories of others who healed or controlled the disease symptoms through methods such as meditation, food, and lifestyle changes.

> The act of getting out of our own way can be the difference between viewing the situation through one lens or allowing multiple lenses to educate you on the "best way to heal" ... *for you.*

Healing is not achieved from just one angle; healing begins when we are curious about how we feel and make connections to prior events. For example, if you are living with celiac disease (a gluten intolerance), and you become sick after eating out, you will immediately assume the restaurant is the cause and cross-contaminated wheat into the meal. This is an obvious correlation, but what happens when the cause of sickness is more subtle?

Healing is a journey, and the first step begins when we become curious about why. Your disease or symptoms today did not occur overnight. Illness happens slowly over time, and then sometimes, hits all at once. In one novel, Ernest Hemingway (1926) described how a person becomes bankrupt. He proclaimed, "Gradually, then suddenly."

If we use that same theory with disease, look back to what you have noticed over the past few years. What foods did you eat, and what toxins were around you? When did you first notice a difference in how you feel? What caused you to go to the doctor?

If I had not remained curious, I would have never explored food as medicine, become aware of heavy metal toxicity, or learned from doctors who have healed diseases unconventionally. The act of being curious is difficult because it leads us into the unknown. You wonder what you will find or if you will need to change your lifestyle and habits.

A lot may have changed when you or a loved one were diagnosed. I am simply suggesting remaining curious and open to the possibilities of healing from all angles. This will lead to new ways of thinking and self-discovery. I encourage you to follow the paths you encounter, and explore what feels good, bringing possibility and joy. This may come in the form of someone who provides support and an empathetic ear. You may follow a thread of releasing your fear through therapy, dance, meditation, or laughter.

There is no right or wrong answer, there is no right or perfect way. Embrace what is working for you because your life is about *you*. For example, the act of reading this book could be your first step to letting go. This first step could lead you to another step and then another. Keep following your joy and intuition and experiment with feeling both mentally and physically better, as well as determining what "feeling better" means to you and what works for you in order to feel better.

Chapter 3 Exercise
What Do You Value?

What do you value? Do you value honesty, laughter, joy, accuracy? This short list only includes four example values from a long list of more than ninety that I have created on my website.

Please visit www.identityofhealth.com and look at the list of values. Then, mark the top twenty values for you.

I encourage you not to overthink your decision. Go with your gut. When you read each value, think about its true meaning. Then, evaluate how it feels inside your body.

Once you select your top twenty, wait five minutes, make a cup of tea, then refine your list. Narrow it down to your top ten.

Once you have your list of ten, there are two more steps:

Reflect on your list of ten. I am sure some stand out more than others. Perhaps a few are similar. Refine your list of ten to your top five.

Once you have your top five, take the important last step: *Select your top three*.

These top three are your soul's core Values. They demonstrate what is important to you. They are your North Star, guiding you as you rise above your disease.

Take your time making these lists. Sit in a quiet space and close your eyes. Begin imagining a future where you are healthy. What are you doing, feeling, and being?

You have a choice, and that choice can be addressed with one question: "What do I value?"

Your fear and worry are choices that can and will be justified, whether you decide to be considered a *survivor* or not. It is okay, either way you choose. I know which choice I want for you, but I do not have to live with your choice. You do.

Chapter 4

Envisioning Something New & Support

"A wise man should consider that health is the greatest of human blessings and learn how by his own thought to derive benefit from his illnesses."

– Hippocrates, *The Aphorisms of Hippocrates*

Crash Course on MS

I sat in the neurologist's office with fear. All I knew and understood at the time was that MS left people in wheelchairs, on their way to an early death. As I listened to my life changing drastically in front of me, I was frozen in fear and the loss of my old self. The words said and options presented were not given time to settle in, as I sat in shock. My experience of recovering from the TIAs and a paralyzed leg told me to ask questions and not commit to anything yet.

I knew fear was a terrible place to be in while making a decision. I was told if I did not move ahead with the medication, which included a 2.5-hour intravenous injection, I would be visiting the doctor again, but in a wheelchair. The doctor did not intend or want to elicit fear, but at this point, it was impossible to avoid.

At a time like this, we have a choice: To follow the treatment the doctor suggests—which may come with risks and side effects—or to explore other options. At this point, it is difficult to hear anything else due to the noise you may hear from doctors, family, and more importantly, yourself. I had been afraid in a doctor's office before and knew how easy it was to say "yes" to their suggestions.

I leaned on the brief research I had done regarding using food as medicine, and I felt hope that there was another option. This was all I needed to make another choice. I knew this other choice had to start immediately, and I was the only one who could prescribe my own path to feel better and control the symptoms of what I was diagnosed with.

I had begun paying attention to what I ate and how I felt with certain foods. I followed rabbit trails of "food as medicine" ideas and research and began studying soil health and toxins in our food streams. I was stepping onto a path that would shape my life with many ups and downs.

I had some things against me. I was not a medical doctor, but I could read, seek help, and educate myself regarding what was happening to me.

There is a scene from the movie *Good Will Hunting* where Matt Damon's character is engaged in banter at a bar with a Harvard student. With the wittiness that can only be scripted and executed in movies, Matt explained to the Harvard guy that his same education could be achieved with a library card.

I realize and understand there is more achieved when attending any university, but I did not have the time or resources to receive formal education on the matter, so I had to pursue educating myself to control MS unconventionally. I began reading books, reviewing medical journals, and studying how others had controlled MS through diet, stress reduction, and exercise.

One, in particular, was Dr. Terry Wahls, a neurologist out of Iowa City, who was diagnosed with Primary Progressive MS. It was a similar prognosis as mine, and she managed to go from being bedridden to riding a bicycle in less than a year. Education and understanding the disease in greater detail brought confidence in my decision and began to shift my mindset on what I could do to have this disease not drastically alter my life.

At this moment, something changed in me regarding the pedestal I had placed doctors on for all these years. People listen to and hold doctors on a pedestal, which has been referenced as the "God Complex." These two egos—your perceptions of your past and the doctors' expert opinions—blend to limit your perceived choices.

For many people, a doctor = God. At least, to some degree.

For me, I had put my trust into a doctor and realized that doctors did not have all the answers. They were just like me but with extensive medical training and education. Doctors, as great as they are, make mistakes, because they are human. They heal and fix based on their training, and oftentimes, it works as planned and many people are saved. For this, I am extremely grateful.

But what happens when they do not know the exact treatment or a solution to a patient's ailment? Due to most people's history of growing up with doctors, it can be extremely difficult to question them, for some people. For example, imagine you grew up with your family only seeking medical expertise from the top doctors. No other healing modalities like food, energy healers, acupuncture, or self-care were ever discussed as you grew into the adult you are. Imagine you become seriously ill with a disease. This disease has few treatments, and all the doctors you saw did not have answers or solutions.

In my situation, which was very similar to the one I just asked you to imagine, the veil of the Doctor = God syndrome had lifted. I was determined not to let my choices be limited.

A Circle of Trust—Overcoming Doubt/Building Confidence

My decision not to take the drug and to go against the neurologist's advice was met with doubt and fear from those around me. When I spoke to friends and family regarding what I was doing to control and halt my MS, I could feel, and sometimes see, their eyes roll. I could hear the tone in their voices and see the facial expression I call "the look." I was sensitive and aware of "the look," so I was keen to identify it. "The look" consisted of doubt, questions, and apprehension of the choice I was making. "The look" left me with my own doubt about my choice.

However, I had researched that MS could be addressed with a healthy diet—avoiding toxins and replacing them with key nutrients—meditation to reduce stress, and exercise to keep muscles active.

As I soon found out, I had to be careful about who I told and what I said. In the early stages of educating myself and taking the steps toward controlling MS, I was easily swayed, and doubt crept in.

Doubt was *dangerous*.

It either slowed my momentum and actions to feel better, or it left me feeling afraid again, which only brought stress. This fear pulled me away from making the positive choices that made me feel better. The doubt had me leaning toward the easy choices—not doing anything, thinking that I did not have a choice, and/or becoming a victim of my circumstances.

I remember going to a restaurant with friends, and as everyone ordered big, juicy hamburgers on fresh buns with sides of French fries, I had to confidently order food that met my dietary choices. I received looks and comments only friends can deliver, and you love them for it. I knew that if I was not confident in myself and the choices I was making, these comments and jokes would stop all the work I had been doing.

The looks and comments became the first realization that halting MS was going to be about choosing what I thought and taking action. The habits and choices I made would either strengthen my resolve or keep me in a pattern that led to disease. I grounded myself in the reality that *I love me*. Then, the choice was solely for me, not them.

As I heard the noise from myself and friends, I had four options to choose from that day:

1. Say okay, follow suit, and order the hamburger and fries on a gluten bun.

2. Proclaim proudly that I do not eat those foods and explain why. (This scenario does not typically go well, and I do not recommend doing this.)

3. Not eat, become upset, and play victim, with the outcome that I would not be invited out to lunch again.

4. Chose to order what I wanted and be happy. Yes, I altered the menu a bit, which the restaurant was happy to do. Then, I could eat and move on with self-pride.

I chose the fourth option, confidently, and moved on without giving it another thought or excuse. I had made the decision, and I was going to take my health into my own hands. My desire to control MS and feel better became my strength against fear.

My choice did not mean I didn't have doubt or the desire for something different. I had made a choice—*that I did not want to give MS any control of my life*. My choice to alter what I ate was stronger than the quick satisfaction or fleeting feeling of being accepted. The choice to live this way did not make me feel any better about the doubt and fear.

The doubt and fear that creeps in tests your decision, and ultimately, the choice of What You Want. Your friends, family, colleagues, doctors, and whomever else you talk to about using an alternate route of healing begin to test the realities of *Who You Are* and *the choices you make*.

Through this, I reminded myself that my friends, family, and others are not me. They do not have to experience the effects of MS. I do.

My family and friends did not have a doctor explain a diagnosis, then attach a label to this diagnosis, and with it, the fear that immediately followed. I knew if I took the feedback as judgment and became upset, I was only hurting myself further, with stress and anger. During this time, I tried to see it from a different angle and walk a mile in my friends' shoes. I attempted to understand what they were feeling.

Your family and friends love you, and you are as much a part of their lives as they are of yours. As much as your friends and family want to help, you have dropped a "bomb" on them, in the form of your disease, which I found leaves them scared, too. They are only trying to help, the best way they know how.

Those around you may not be trained or experienced with helping a friend through the frightening diagnosis you received. Their only experience and knowledge of dealing with frightening information may come from movies, news sources, books, and maybe first-hand experience. They often do not understand that your mindset through this situation is critical. My grandfather said it best: "I am asking questions and giving you a hard time because I love you. If I did not say anything, then you would have something to worry about."

Building a Support System That Supports You

I have empathy for anyone helping a loved one through healing and/or battling any disease. I could see my kids, who are my biggest believers and pillars of support, become lost at times for what to say or how to act. I began to realize that they needed my support, patience, and love as much as I needed theirs.

As someone who had their life changed with one phone call, I had to remember that my children's lives were changed too. They did not need to hear my fear as anger and depression. They needed a source of strength, which starts with being vulnerable and open. Standing on a strong foundation meant being open to listening, learning, and asking about their fears with no judgment. Listening to them was as healing for me as it was for them. These conversations enhanced our understanding of each other, and I was beginning to feel genuinely *heard*.

At this time, there was not much I could control, other than my thoughts, my exercise routine, and the foods I ate. I remembered a story from *Anthony William in his book Medical Medium:* A woman who was bedridden became paralyzed from the neck down, due to her illness. All she wanted was to walk again, or at least, to be able to hug her kids and laugh. As she laid there, she realized that all she could control was her thoughts and her prayers. She began asking the angels around her for help. After some time, she could feel her fingers, then slowly wiggle them, which eventually led to walking again, shocking all the doctors and everyone else. If she had approached the situation as a victim, thinking "woe is me," if she had listened to those around her, she most likely would still be in the hospital bed.

Belief to Heal

Through these moments remember, *you always have a choice.*

During your journey of taking your health into your own hands, what you tell yourself and what you Believe is *critical*. Your thoughts are stronger than anything you may encounter from others.

I have one friend who—when asked how he is doing—always states that he is "Magnificent!" When he says it, you believe him. He decided, "This is who I am, and this is how I want to feel." He makes a choice about how his life will be dictated, no matter what happens.

The people around you generally have the best intentions. They do not want to make your life more difficult. Their intention is not to seed doubt in your mind, prove that they are right, or give the mighty-yet-bullshit statement, "I told you so." In moments of conflict or disagreement with the people around you, most people tend to lead with their own perceptions and past experiences, both verbal and non-verbal. In these moments, we look at the other person's facial expressions and the tone of their voice, and we begin filling in the blanks of what we *think* they mean. Often, we are incorrect.

All of us have experienced situations when we feel the other person does not have the best intentions. During times like these or in times of doubt, knowing What You Want and the choices you made to get there can give you strength. You are saving your own life and well-being. It is both a choice to save yourself, and it is the most important work you can ever do.

When situations or feelings happen that are not nurturing or supportive, you can either allow it to affect your day, or you can let it go, immediately. I choose not to allow anything anyone says or how I feel about a situation to have control over me. I choose to confine it, think of it as "just a single moment."

Although this statement may seem simple, doubt can seem impossible to avoid. I want to introduce an exercise for you to use in doubtful moments. (We'll go further with this exercise in a later chapter.)

Chapter 4 Exercise

Exercise for Doubtful Moments

In your journal, you have begun to explore Who You Are and your Values. Building on these, I would like you to begin thinking about What You Want for yourself. Not just stating the external desires like money, a house, or other material goods, but I would like you to state how you want to *feel* when you receive these.

For example, you might envision yourself receiving your desires and write something like, "I want to feel stable and balanced when I finally have my dream house and dream car," or "I want to experience love and joy in my life."

Now, in your journal, write down what you want and how you would like to feel once you have received what you want.

Imagine what you are doing when you feel this way. Where are you? Who is with you? What does the ground feel like? Can you feel the breeze on your face? What does it smell like?

For example, I might write, "I want to feel pain free and joyful, and I want my walking to be stable and enjoyable."

When I write this, I am setting the intention of how I am being, *feeling as if I have already received my desire*, based on who I am and my Values and how these make me feel.

When you write out your desired feelings, acting as if you have received what you have desired, you set that intention. How does this *feel*?

The feeling of setting the intention is where creation begins, which we will explore in later chapters. You have begun building the strength and resolve needed to rise above the noise you hear. When we act and imagine as if it has already happened, no matter your current external situation, we are setting the stage for our desire to become present in our current lives.

As our Belief grows to our desire, we let go to allow the amazing to surprise us.

Support

During the times when doubt and fear are the noisiest, most pressing feelings, support is critical. You need a team to advise, support, and help you heal. They are there to help you succeed. I recommend that you do not try to chase your health or success alone.

This support and healing team should be made of people who understand the desires and wants that you have written in your journal. They should also be aware of your worries, and you should understand theirs.

I could not and would not rely on my healing team for education, nor do I advise that someone leave the decision-making up to them. For me, I saw my support team more as an advisory board or council.

It is your responsibility to identify your support team, ask their permission, and help them be an incredible team for you. Be the leader I know you are for yourself and others.

As you create your support team, there are important steps to take as you set your intentions to heal.

First, make a list of who is on your team—family, therapist, coach, support groups, and friends. Choose individuals who are supportive, empathetic, and willing to walk a mile in your shoes. Choose people who lovingly point out when you are not following your Values.

Second, take time to sit with them and clearly define where you are going and what your journey means to you. Share your plan and tell them how you are going to reach your goals. Show them the areas where you'll have difficulty and talk with them about how they can help you rise above your challenges.

This doesn't need to be a long conversation or set up like an executive board meeting built with agendas and presentations. It can be short and quick, something that can be repeated or explained at any time to anyone.

During this time, be open. Listen to your team members' opinion or concerns. It does not mean you have to take their advice. Their perspective may contain more information and an idea you have not explored.

If the individual does not believe in what you are doing, that is okay. You now know how to take their looks, comments, and advice. You know where they stand and what type of support they are willing to offer. By having this conversation, you can remove the labels and stories that you put on the situations in your life and your interpretation of them.

Third, keeping your healing team informed is important, and they want it too. I began by sharing success stories, keeping team members up to speed about how I was progressing and the knowledge I gained. My updates involved having friends over for dinner for casual conversation, or the occasional phone call to ask about them and not about me.

Once I began communicating regularly with my team members, my mind shifted to a focus on how I was going to support my team members. That shift in focus became better than simply talking more about my situation.

If you have ever read Dr. Robert Cialdini's work in his book Influence, he describes how one of the core principles of influence is reciprocity. The basic principle states that if I help people achieve what they want, they will have a desire to help me achieve what I want.

Once I removed myself from the burden of "having to update someone" and shifted my focus to "How can I help them?", my team became more supportive and interested in how they could help me. I did not want my team members feeling like they now had a job, a job that required them to read and address my updates. Nor did I want to give myself the task or burden of having to provide regular updates. I wanted this to be a collaboration that was fueled by genuine care and concern for one another.

Your team loves you, and you give them the opportunity to find more meaning and joy in their lives through supporting you during your difficult time.

Chapter 4 Exercise

Putting Words into Practice with Mantras/Communication Skills

I have a mantra I tell myself when I begin to feel the swell of doubt or frustration that stems from my perception or reaction to a negative feeling or situation. At these moments, I tell myself, "I am the highest and best for me and all involved."

This may be a difficult phrase to digest, especially when these moments have touched an especially sensitive trigger. If the triggering situation is the result of a comment made from a spouse, family, close friend, or parent, it can be difficult to allow this feeling to drift past you, like a leaf in a river.

In a situation when you are triggered, talk to them directly about it. The hardest part about having this conversation is stopping and taking the first leap of faith. If this conversation is too difficult, look back at What You Want and how you want to be supported. Begin by sharing with them how their statement made you feel. Share how they could best support your journey to control your disease.

Everyone around you is part of your healing team. Like a good coach or leader, you have to help them know how to support you best. It is your responsibility to build your support team and teach them what you need and where you are going. If you have new dietary restrictions, for example, tell them about your new diet. Let them know how they can help.

Let people around you know how best to support you and address situations quickly when you feel less than confident.

Having these conversations means that you must approach them with an open mind. You must listen to and address all situations with love. Remember, the people on your team are scared too, and they may feel lost with how best to help you. I found that when I intentionally built my healing team, they became my biggest cheerleaders and believers, oftentimes helping me rise above my own negative self-talk.

Conclusion

There is a lot in my life that I *have* to do, or that I am *required* to do. For example, I *have to* pay attention to my family, my business, my hobbies, my friendships, and my new habits. Do not get me wrong—these are joys in my life, and I love doing them, most of the time.

Controlling my symptoms and feeling better with a disease is *not* one of these joys, but I had to change my perspective if I wanted to control my MS. I did not want my healing to be "just another task" for me or others. To alleviate this burden on myself and others, I had to make a choice: Was I going to be vulnerable and ask for help?

Over time, this choice became easier, and I removed my mask of fear and shame. I let others into my fear, shame, joy, and life, by becoming vulnerable. When I did that, updating my team and helping them no longer became a task, it became a way of life—joyful and effortless. Once I let go and allowed others to help, once I felt safe that everyone around me was on the same page, different doors opened and additional encouragement arrived in my life. These doors opened because I had clearly stated my intention, imagining that it had already happened. I was open to seeing things from the area of possibility and not scarcity. As my thoughts opened these doors, I was available and present to explore these new options and surrender to the possible change.

If I had left myself in a state of fear, judgment, and anger, I would have been closed off from learning life's important lessons; in every moment, I would have become a victim. When I became a student who was ready, multiple teachers appeared. Not all teachers told me what I wanted to hear, and at times, they told me what I needed to hear. Through these interactions, I found myself becoming more confident and supported in my choices.

I took the "looks" and the comments of both support and doubt as comical or as coming from a place of love; I took them as the push that I needed to keep going.

All of this was not going to happen accidentally or simply because I wanted it. My healing team needed to know how, when, and why to support me. I needed to know where I was headed, so I could become more confident, the leader I needed to be, taking action when needed. I acted on how I wanted to be and had loving conversations with everyone around me.

> It is your choice whether you declare
> What You Want and let others encourage you or
> whether they leave you feeling less than enough.
> From the bottom of my heart,
> I know you are enough and stronger than
> you may give yourself credit for.

Chapter 5

Who are You?

"To be yourself in a world that is constantly trying to make you something else is the greatest accomplishment."

– Ralph Waldo Emerson, *Essays*

Who I Was & Who I Became

I left the house early on a cold October morning to run ten miles and try to relieve stress that had been building at work. As I ran down a narrow back-country road with woods on my left and a cornfield on my right, I noticed movement in the sky about 200 yards away. As I got closer, the movement was revealed as a group of more than 100 small blackbirds pouring out of a wooded ravine and into a tree on the edge of the road.

As one group entered the tree, another group of more than 100 careened out of the tree and into the cornfield. As I stood there for over fifteen minutes, watching this dance, I was in awe of the beauty I was witnessing. I loved these moments when training— witnessing and experiencing little moments of life that seemed only for me.

These are the moments I miss, and letting go of my old sense of self became a challenge. I was regularly reminded of what I had done in my life and who I had made myself into. I remembered how I felt and the moments of joy and pride when I became an All-American Triathlete. How I lost eighty-five pounds, turning long runs into my moments of Zen.

I wanted them all back, and the depression of losing who I once was became a bigger challenge than my symptoms of MS. I was living in a past that could not be lived again, no matter how bad I wanted it. I stopped seeing the gift of these moments, remembering instead the lessons they taught me.

I held on to my past so tightly that it kept me from moving forward to the new life I was creating. It was easy to allow the thoughts and desires of my past to keep me in a reality that could not exist anymore. I was so focused on my past that I could not see who I was today in the Present Moment.

It was hard to imagine who I wanted to become, difficult not to be defined by a diagnosis. It was easier to remain in my self-pity party, mourning my past. It was justified by me and others. I realized during this time that I had a choice: Continue living in a past that brought depression and loss that I could do nothing about, or define who I wanted to be with joy and love.

My view of the MS diagnosis at this time began to shift; I began to see it as the gift that it was. I was given an opportunity to become someone new. To dig deeper into my sense of Self and wake up to my incredible soul. This next phase of my life was an opportunity to redefine who I was and who I wanted to be. We all have an opportunity to become who we are meant to be, every moment of every day. A diagnosis of any kind is an opportunity to do that.

When I was diagnosed with MS, I had a choice of whether I adopted this new label or not. This new label could have drastically changed my perspective of what I think I could do and not do. Yes, some diagnoses cause you to change drastically, due to pain, lack of mobility, or another event. They are all very real, and in some cases, the only thing we can control is who we think we are and what we tell ourselves, leading with our limiting beliefs or possibility.

Identity: Self-Image, Self-Esteem, Ideal Self

Our identity of Who We Think We Are is a foundation we stand on; it grounds us and provides a sense of security. A strong sense of Self also provides peace of knowing where we are going, our desires, and where the Present Moment is leading us. The foundation of our identity happens when we are grounded in who we think we are and when we are aware of our sense of Self. We have a foundation to return to when times are difficult. We are grounded in Awareness and have the opportunity to love ourselves under any condition. This grounding is an anchor; it is true North; it is home.

We shape and craft our lives because of what we want, not for anyone else. It was not until my reality was shaken and the rug pulled out from under me that I realized how important this was. With a phone call from a doctor, a shovelful of snow, and hitting the side of a wooden box, my sense of Self was tested. Who I thought I was came crashing down abruptly, with no warning. My habits, my way of life, my joy, and the sense of Self that I created was not paid attention to or given importance, until it was gone.

Humanist psychologist Carl Rogers identified three contributing components to the development of the sense of Self: self-image, self-esteem, and the Ideal Self.

As summarized by McLeod (2014), this sense of Self has been studied by many, who have found that the concepts of Who We Think We Are begin developing as early as three years of age. We begin to think, "I am a boy," or "I am a girl." We think, "I have red hair and blue eyes." Thoughts like these create our self-image.

This developing sense of Self begins to craft what we wear and what we do as a child. Do you play with trucks or dolls? What sports do you play? What do you watch on TV? At a young age, people around us either reinforce our sense of self or attempt to sway us in a specific way.

Take a moment to remember what you can from your early childhood—preschool days, if possible. Can you recall the positive feedback you received?

We all have one inherent specific desire during this time, and it is to be loved and accepted. When we are accepted with positive feedback, we tend to continue the activities that are rewarded and where we feel love. When we do not feel the love that we desire, we do not continue the behavior, or we change our behavior to receive acceptance and love.

As we progress into early adolescence and teen years, we develop our sense of self with our self-esteem and "the Ego." We might think: "I am fat," or "I am popular," or "I am athletic." This begins to shape the internal labels that we self-adopt from external feedback or our constant self-talk.

We have not lost our core desire for love and acceptance, but our worlds have expanded past our parents and family and into friends and societal pressures.

As these labels become more ingrained and tied to our sense of Self, we try to mold them to what we Believe is the Ideal Self and what others want. The Ideal Self is developed based on what we see and observe, our experiences, the outside world, our perceptions, and feedback, both positive and negative.

I remember making choices at the age of ten, based on what I thought others wanted. I made choices for myself not just on what I wanted but what I thought would be accepted by others. We have an ancestral desire that was wired into us at birth and developed over thousands of years. As humans, if we were part of a group, it meant safety and survival. If we were cast out, separated from the group and alone, it meant a possible death.

Today, the case is not as severe as it was thousands of years ago, but we have not yet evolved past this ancestral desire of love and acceptance. Today, if we feel that we were not accepted by our peers, it can lead to a feeling of being cast out, and fear quickly follows. I remember being a twelve-year-old kid, wanting to be liked by my friends. I was overweight and could not run as fast as my friends or throw a ball as far. Due to this, I was not picked for sports. I did not feel accepted, which led to depression and a deep desire to fit in. I was looking for ways to gain approval and be seen as important.

I was willing to change my sense of Self to be accepted. These labels and new identity I crafted were dictated by how I viewed myself and what I told myself, even if the voice was negative. As I developed into puberty, this negative sense of self was reinforced by those around me, and the negative label and lack of self-worth grew. These labels that I identified with reinforced my mindset and negative self-talk, which led to anger and depression.

These negative labels or self-perception— "the Ego"—shows itself outwardly when you act out in an attempt to be significant and noticed. This outward appearance can show up as drinking, drugs, crime, or at the least, wearing a mask and pretending to be a perfect perception of Self. As we develop, the mask or actions we take can lead to stress, which can perpetuate depression and a feeling like we are lost.

The scenario described above is a possible outcome that you might identify with or not. As you think about your past and create Awareness of the moments that shaped Who You Are, you have an opportunity to continue living with that perception or not. When the perception of Who We Think We Are leads to long-term unmitigated depression or stress, it can cause health issues. If we are aware of what happened and why, then we have an opportunity to change.

This change can be frightening, as you step into an unknown future, but it is your choice to move forward or not. You have already taken steps to change your self-identity and shape yourself into the ideal that you desire. When we are diagnosed with a disease or other medical challenge, our sense of Self could have drastically changed. Without a strong identity, we can feel lost and continue to spiral into depression and feelings of loss.

Breaking Down & Rebuilding the Self-Image

Our identity and perception of Who We Are—athletic, attractive, smart, detail-oriented, afraid of change, ugly, stupid etc.—are all labels we have decided to adopt. No one has forced these labels on us or told us, "This is the way it has to be." These labels, whether filled with the possibility of life or the feeling of not being enough, either promote our Ideal Self or diminish it.

A positive sense of Self leads us toward possibility, people, and positive choices that ripple outwardly. A negative sense of Self leads to stress, depression, and fear, and may eventually lead to illness or dis-ease.

> How we think about ourselves becomes a self-fulfilling prophecy. What we tell ourselves becomes the reality that we experience.

Identity & Choice

Who We Think We Are and our perception of Self is right. It is very difficult or impossible for someone else to change how we view our sense of Self. This decision is 100 percent your choice, and there is no right or wrong answer. This choice is either going to leave you with an I-am-going-to-beat-this attitude, or it will leave you with fear. Our choice is reflected in what we think, what we say, and the labels we adopt. Our sense of Self can leave us with an I-can-do-it-and-will-try belief, or it can leave us with a belief that we are victims of circumstance and impossibility.

> The difference between someone who thinks they can and someone who thinks they cannot is driven by a sense of Self. Our thoughts lead us to our daily choices and actions.

There are many stories of people achieving the impossible and many others who became a victim of their circumstances. Our identities and sense of who we Believe we are either keep us trying with hope and possibility, or they leave us with feelings that we "can't" or "it is impossible." If our self-image and identities are negative and leave us feeling trapped, it can lead to stress and a sense of not being good enough.

What if, during an unexpected abrupt change—like the diagnosis of a disease—your new label or self-perception was met with a positive sense of Self? Could your positive sense of Self lead you to possibility and the opportunity to heal what you were diagnosed with?

Defining Yourself on Your Own Terms

Our health and the beliefs around our health are foundational aspects that define us. We have an opportunity to stop a diagnosis or current state of being from defining us. We can choose to define it.

There is a motivational speaker by the name of Nick Vujicic, who was born with Tetra-amelia syndrome, which is a rare disorder characterized by the absence of arms and legs. His parents never let him use it as a handicap or limitation. He went on to have a family, become a painter, and skydive, along with many other things. He has also motivated many audiences to rise above any limitation. If his parents did not help develop the mindset of possibility, would he have completed everything that he has? He knew who he was and what he wanted.

So, who are you?

You may have received a diagnosis or had your perception of Who You Were removed. Who you think you were and what you used to be able to do is being challenged, or in some cases, it has been eradicated. Due to this, we are required or being challenged to change and adapt to a new paradigm of Who We Think We Are.

The first step is to address this moment of change. Your past is not meant to be forgotten, ignored, or more importantly, dwelled on; it is meant for you to learn from it. For some, answering the questions of Who You Are is very easy, and for others, it can be difficult. What is happening in your life right now may be forcing you to address it.

Chapter 5 Exercise
Changing the Perception of Self

Below is a small first step if you desire to change a negative mindset and negative perception of Self.

First, do not take this change lightly or think of it as a daunting task where you have to lose or give up anything. Oftentimes, we think of what we *cannot* do instead of thinking about what we *can* do. Change can be more frightening than our own death, and the concept of changing who you think you are may leave you wanting to close the book now and never pick it up again. Before you make a choice and tell yourself that you *cannot*, I would like to tell you a story.

Story of John

I have a good friend by the name of John who has decided to beat cancer. In order to beat cancer and spend his life with his wife, watching his kids grow up, he had to make a choice. His choice to try led him to review how he lives his life, how he views himself, and the choices he makes. Cancer left him with a different perspective.

His cancer diagnosis and dealing with cancer created a new perception of how he lives life with his loved ones. These thoughts aided him in making different choices. These choices and a new loving perspective led him to chase life, to live life *now*. Cancer helped John realize that he did not have time to live life thinking of *someday*. He could not just stand by with hope and be a victim to what was happening in his life.

As he stares at his own mortality daily, John's perception of self and his fear of cancer are perpetuated with every scan and doctor's appointment. Thankfully, he is now in remission, and every doctor appointment leaves him with clear scans.

One day, he handed me a hat with the letters RFN on the front. He explained to me that he made the choice to live life to its fullest—"RFN." *Right Fucking Now!*

John's inspirational story as a witness to a beautiful life, fully living in the Present Moment, began with one choice. This choice led him to another and then another. He did not worry about the past, as he realized that his life *was* right now.

It was a time to love and start healing and living RFN.

Self-Talk

One of the best ways to start is to explore what we tell ourselves, to become aware of what we think. Exploring our self-perception can be a difficult road. As we dig into our sense of Self, we uncover some aspects that we are not proud of or that are difficult to understand and deal with.

Think of these discoveries or realizations as roadblocks to getting where you want to be. Also, give yourself a break and remember to love yourself deeply and give gratitude that you are changing your thoughts and your life *now*.

For example, if we are on a road trip and the only road going to our destination is blocked by debris, and no one is around, we would get out of our car and move what is blocking us. Depending on its size, we may require assistance from others. Moving a large log with four people is much easier than moving it alone.

When we are diagnosed with a disease, we are given the label of *having* something—cancer, MS, another autoimmune condition, etc. This label may require changes in our life or the loss of who we thought we were. This loss may lead to fear, making us hold on tightly to our past, which is a roadblock. Through our challenges, we realize the old ways we thought and lived are not supporting our healing.

We may want to heal and get past this label of our diagnosis, in order to live and survive. We know where we want to go, but our strong desire to hold on to our past (because it is comfortable and known) becomes the roadblock or mental debris. Depending on the size and impact of our concept of "who we once were," removing this debris can be difficult, but it is not impossible.

> I found that Awareness of the debris allowed me
> to take steps to remove it, piece by piece.
> Removing the roadblock does not have to be done
> alone, which is the good part.

Allow and be open to help; it will require you to become vulnerable and ask for help. This can be done with friends, family, or from the healing and support team mentioned in the previous chapter. This team should understand who you are, where you are going, and what needs to be removed. Having confidants who understand what you are trying to achieve, people who listen and hear you, will be a lifesaving gift.

Chapter 5 Exercise

Reviewing Last Week

Take a moment to look back on the last week. Remember, there is no judgment. It just *is*—no right, no wrong.

- What happened?
- When did you feel alone?
- What was the encouragement or fear you told yourself?
- Did people you meet brighten your day, or did you feel they reinforced your negative sense of self?
- What were you thinking about yourself?
- Did you use "absolute" words like *always* or *never*?

When we think in absolute terms, we take away our options and choices. Yes, limiting your choices is a safer way to exist, but it can also be a dangerous way of existence, especially when it comes to your health.

Understanding Who You Are and working through mental roadblocks may seem like a one-person sport. I have found that when I explored my sense of Self alone, I stayed on my known similar path. When I sought help from a therapist, coach, and an empathetic friend for encouragement, I became aware of my blind spots. I could not see it all by myself.

When I realized I could rely on this support, I tended to stay on my path and remove blockages in my way in order to heal.

External support can help you be aware of your ingrained, automatic language. Once I shone a light on my shadows, the shadows disappeared, and I became aware of my limiting thoughts.

After doing this work, taking the time to understand Who I Was and What I Wanted to Be, I began building a foundation of "I can." Just like the old sense of self you held on to, your new healing and positive Self will become your new identity and strong healing foundation.

After this work, there was nothing that anyone could say that would shake me from the core of who I think I am, or to get in my way of feeling better and healing.

Chapter 5 Exercise

Exploring Who You Are

If you are exploring the question of Who You Are, start by using a sheet of blank paper in your journal. The questions below will push you to explore the core of Who You Are.

Ask yourself these questions and record your answers. Write, draw pictures, or jot your answers in whatever form resonates with you.

Take twenty minutes and write down what first comes to mind.

- What did I once love about who I was?
    - Hint: It starts with *used to*, for example, *I used to run faster than anyone else.*
- What did I tell people I did when asked?
    - Hint: It starts with *I am*: *I am a father. I am a salesman* (or any other profession, etc.).
- What are my adopted identities?
    - Hint: These are probably how other people would describe you: mother, father, grandmother, etc.; athlete (include which sport); smart; loving; detailed-oriented; etc.
- What is the one thing that I enjoy doing every day?

- What do I miss?
- What is one of the funniest moments of my life that I can recall? (Take your time.)
- What is one of the most humbling moments of my life that I can recall? (Take your time.)

You are making a list of Who You Are, *now*! Any language that does not promote your feeling of greatness, simply cross it out. You are now aware of what your negative inner voice might be saying.

What did you find out?

Did you discredit or lessen the impact of what you wrote? For example, if you wrote down, "I am a musician," then said to yourself, "It was not that big of a deal," or "I really only knew a few songs..." you are lessening the impact and greatness of yourself.

- What did you *feel* when you wrote those answers?
- Did you feel *happy* or *sad*, *encouraged* or *fearful*, etc.?
- Did you feel *energized* by any of the memories?

We are going to pay attention to these feelings as they begin to bring you closer to the core of Who You Are.

Can you drill further into any of the questions and answers?

Write down a pattern or theme you may have recognized.

Exercise Part 2—Exploring Who You Are

As you are becoming aware of the patterns and greatness of you and how you feel around these, it is time to craft Who You Want to Be.

Using the words you identified, write a one-sentence statement of who you are now. Shorter is better!

For example:

Starting with **I AM**: I am a father of two; I am fully healed; I am Love, Joy; I am an author, speaker, coach, healer, passionate fisherman, lover of beautiful sunsets, kind, and funny.

Your sentence can be anything. Make every word count!

Practice and experiment with Who You Are. Take your time practicing it. Write it down a few times and share it with loved ones you trust.

- How does it feel?
- Do you Believe your "I am" statement(s)?
- What would it take for you to Believe and live your "I am" statement(s)?

> You may not Believe your new identity at first, so give it time and change it as needed.

Final Thoughts/Conclusion

You have not changed, and you are still the incredible person you were before all this happened. The way you approach or view your life now may have changed. But these changes can be positive, if we let them be. However, change requires us to let go of the old, in order to receive our new sense of Self.

Your "I am" statement changes and evolves, so keep updating it. Remember to use words that lift you up and make you feel good about yourself, not dim your light. Love yourself and use these positive statements about yourself to begin making different choices.

> You have started to walk the path of Self-discovery, which can lead you to the habits and actions to create the results you want. You are

worth every word and positive piece of
encouragement you can tell yourself.

There is a difference between those who rise above the negative self-talk and encourage themselves with joy and love. The difference is possibility and knowing that they can.

Chapter 6

What Do You Want?

"The journey of a thousand miles begins with one step."

– Lao Tzu, *Tao Te Ching*

I was a terrible student in high school and in college. I was more interested in getting noticed and being accepted. I rarely thought about what I wanted or what I was going to do after college. Not knowing what I wanted to do in my life and something to strive for left me floating aimlessly.

My lack of direction left me caring just enough to give more than the minimum effort. I remember sitting in algebra class in high school as concepts and formulas floated past me. As I tried to absorb the material and understand the concepts, my mind often drifted. I found out the hard way (with poor grades) that letting your mind drift in algebra is a bad idea. Teachers would refer to this as "daydreaming," but I saw it as lack of caring. I could not see why I was learning the material. I wanted something more, and my time at school was often experienced as boredom.

As high school unfolded, my lack of direction and poor grades led to barely being accepted into Marquette University. Without good habits, my approach to my college education had little to no focus. In college, I remember dreaming about working and wanting only the physical objects: car, house, money, etc.

I later realized that this was what an immature twenty-year-old man wants. As the four years of college came to an end, I was still fifteen credits short of graduating. My fiancée at the time was graduating and moving on, and I wanted to be with her. So, I left school and moved to Colorado.

<blockquote style="text-align:center">
All of that could have been avoided
if I answered and gave thought to the question:
What do I want?
</blockquote>

The Negative Thoughts

According to research published in the journal *Nature Communications* in 2020, an average person has more than 6,000 thoughts per day. Of those, **80 percent are negative** and **95 percent are repetitive thoughts**. We live in a perpetual negative thought pattern more than a positive one.

Our mindset during the day has more possibility of leading us toward a feeling of not being good enough. If we allow these thoughts to percolate, they will lead us toward negative behaviors and actions. We binge listen to the negative dialogue in our heads, remembering all the times we made a mistake or said something that was not quite right.

The loud voice in our heads (that only we hear) is relentless. It says awful things like, "You are not good enough. What if you screw up? You know you are not smart enough." Along with a slew of other nasty things.

If this voice were a person, we would commit them to an insane asylum, or at least, have a restraining order against them. Instead, we invite this person in to live with us every minute we are awake. The more we let this negative voice alter our beliefs and perceptions, the voice begins to transfer to our feelings and behaviors. Our behaviors are experienced by ourselves and others as anxiety, stress, and depression. If we let these feelings go on too long, it creates *dis-ease*, or an imbalance, in our bodies.

We make choices every minute of every day regarding what we think, so why do we let our past thoughts and beliefs create this reality for us?

This voice, although terrible at times, does serve a purpose. Our inner negative critic can be an alarm, used to assess risk and danger, as it was intended. But there is a difference between the voice of our inner critic being critical and the voice of an inner mentor who encourages.

An inner mentor is quiet and reminds us to pay attention and love ourselves. The mentor's voice encourages us and tells us when we should slow down. Over time, we can drown out the inner mentor with our inner critic, who mutes the inner voice we need most, the voice that encourages and supports us.

> You have control and choice over *everything* that runs through your thoughts.

Each of us has the choice to listen or not. We have the choice to ask the ultimate question that brings us back to our center and sense of a positive Self.

Are these negative thoughts true?

Our internal voice, negative or not, stems from the labels we give ourselves or that are given to us by others. For many years, while I competed in triathlons, I would hear Ironman Triathletes discuss the fact that Ironman was 70 percent mental. At the time, I told myself and others there was no way this was true!

Ironman competitions consist of a 2.4-mile open-water swim, then a 112-mile bike ride, and then a 26.2-mile run. All must be completed within seventeen hours.

When I completed my first Ironman in 2011, I found the statement about how much mental energy could contribute to a triathlete's success to be correct.

One year before completing the Ironman, I was recovering from a paralyzed leg. I had not run consistently for two years. My past endurance was not helping me, so I leaned on the 70 percent statistic with training.

Your thoughts on whether or not you can achieve a goal leads us to possibility. The Navy SEALs, for example, train under the context that when your mind is telling you that you're "done," you're really only 40 percent done, no matter what you're trying to accomplish.

When we start setting small goals and achieving them, it leads us to another step. When we do this, we utilize a tactic called The Power of 1 Percent Better.

Where in your life are you improving by 1 percent every day?

Often, we set a large goal and think we need to achieve the outcome as fast as possible. In the story of the tortoise and the hare racing each other, I know the result is always the same: The tortoise wins.

Why? Because, as the moral of the story tells us, *Slow and steady wins the race.*

I understood and used the mental aspects of competing, staying positive, listening to my body, and knowing that pain is temporary. Also, I knew that I was a good triathlete, so I enjoyed every aspect of the sport, which helped a lot.

At the time, triathlons were a big part of Who I Was, and being an Ironman is what I wanted. This positive image led me to a feeling that I could—no matter what setback or roadblock I encountered.

My positive outlook led me to train, no matter how bad it hurt, taking small steps. I took the time to build the endurance I needed. Over the course of the year of training, I adjusted my life for whatever new habit I needed to build in order to cross that finish line. I wanted to finish Ironman, achieving a goal that I looked at for eight years, a goal that, at one point, I thought I would never achieve, due to my paralyzed leg three years before.

More importantly, I wanted to know that I was okay. I knew it was going to be my last race. I wanted to be able to say goodbye to triathlons on my terms.

As I ran to the finish line, more than thirteen hours later, I stopped when I was only fifty yards away. Imagine the moment: You have just spent thirteen hours and twenty-one minutes finishing all three of the challenges. You have a crowd of people on both sides of you, screaming and cheering you on. High-fives are being distributed, no matter where you turn. The feelings of accomplishment, pride, and joy of being done flood your emotions.

As I walked toward the finish line, soaking in a moment I knew I would never have again, I felt free. I was not sad or disappointed; I was complete. I had accomplished my goal while overcoming impossible odds.

> All of it started with knowing that I could do it and with knowing what I wanted.

Putting Ego in Check

Addressing our false expectations for ourselves (or Who We Thought We Wanted to Be) is a big step toward defining Who We (*actually*) Want to Be. If we default to doing nothing, no one else will concern themselves with our happiness as much as we should or will as individuals.

When you are healing anything or trying to deal with any change, take one small step. Review your list of Who You Are. Begin remembering that you are enough, and you are awesome, no matter the circumstance. You are being given an opportunity to look deep within yourself. You are a gift, and you are loved by those around you and from above.

More importantly, love yourself. Be grateful for Who You Are. Embrace this love and begin knowing and believing that you *can*. As you look toward What You Want—no matter how big or small—it is a step toward knowing that you *can*. Knowing this helps you establish a foundation for your healing journey.

If we do not take the time to answer these questions and decide what we ultimately want, we can easily be swayed or influenced. The negative or positive voice is always going to be there. When the voice leads us to fear and a sense of not being good enough, it may stop our ability to act or make a decision.

I had a mentor in my life who used to say a phrase that has stuck with me, and I repeat it when my Ego is testing my choices:

> "If I do not decide what I want, someone else will do it for me, and it will suck."

You would not go to a restaurant and let someone order for you. So why would you let someone decide what your life, health, and reason should be?

You are amazing, and you are enough. No matter what you have been diagnosed with or what situation you are in, no matter how bleak, you still have a choice. One of the greatest gifts God gave us was free will. No one can make you do anything; you have a choice. When we are left in fear and have told ourselves, "I am trapped," then it is time to stop, slow down, and remind yourself What You Want.

Love yourself.

If someone does not know who they are and what they want, then yes, the choices seem limited. We are only limited by what we tell ourselves or the limits we accept.

Remain positive. Others do not know your situation. They are not in the doctor's office with you. They do not know your life and what you are truly feeling. Your circumstances may be real, but your friends, family, and other people were not the ones who created them.

If you created your circumstances, then you can change them. I have seen homeless immigrants become millionaires and have met people who have overcome and healed brain cancer, diabetes, and MS.

> We all have a choice, and it becomes clearer when we know what we want.

Labels

Every day you either adopt a new label or reinforce a current one. This label leads to what we tell ourselves, leaves us thinking we can or we can't. Our internal sense of Self and knowledge about Who We Are leads us to What We Want. For example, if you think you are detail oriented and had a positive experience with numbers and specifically accounting, you most likely would move toward accounting as a degree in college. If you truly love accounting, you may move toward advanced studies. Although being difficult for most, you find it rewarding and fun. All because you thought you were detail oriented and good with numbers.

Think of a moment in your life, hobbies you have, and the regular thoughts that lead you down a specific path. Was this path enjoyable? Did you feel confident when exploring it?

In 2017, I was fired from my position and not given a reason. This lack of reason or understanding of why I was fired was unclear. My self-manufactured reason painted a picture of a victim. According to my colleagues at the position, I did nothing wrong; I wasn't accused of harassment or other terrible HR mistakes, and my results were exceeding the goal.

This lack of knowing tore me down daily, because I let it. The only thing that I could do was learn from it. To make matters worse, I was let go less than thirty days before being diagnosed with MS. With both bombs dropped so close to each other, all I felt I could do was wallow in my own self-pity. The situations I experienced at the time felt out of my control.

I remember feeling angry, sad, and lost. I was living with an extremely stressful mindset that there was nothing I could do. I was allowing my situations and those around me to craft my reality of who I thought I was, instead of allowing myself to craft my own reality.

This negative mindset and very real situations left me with a sense of not being good enough. This state of pity was not me, and I knew I had to change now or the road I continued down would lead me to behavior and results with worse consequences. This decision to change what I thought and perception of myself has caused me to grow into the person I am today.

As I look back, I was being challenged on what I believed about myself. During that time of loss and fear, I met with as many people as I could or was mentally able to handle.

One person I was meeting with asked me the question, "What do you want?"

I had never asked myself this question, nor had I ever been asked this question directly. It ended up being the hardest question I have ever answered.

When I looked inward and really thought about what I wanted, I began asking different questions. This seemingly simple question—"What do you want?"—developed my reason for overcoming the negative thoughts I was experiencing. This one simple question led me down a path of inward reflection.

This path is one of Self-discovery, in an attempt to understand ourSelves. Once we start listening to our inner intuitive voice, we are regularly challenged on whether or not we listen to it and what we truly believe about ourSelves. These challenges are not bad but a way for us to continue growing and developing ourselves.

Trusting Your Intuition

> All of us have this voice that resides within us,
> and we make the choice to listen to it or not.

During this time, I remember one of my guides and teachers described "the intuitive 2x4." The "intuitive 2x4" is the little voice in the back of your mind that makes a quiet statement, trying to get your attention.

One day, I was at the grocery store and heard this quiet voice in the back of my mind say, "Make sure you grab some peanut butter."

I ignored the voice and thought, "We do not need peanut butter."

As I walked down the next aisle, the voice came back and said, "Grab some peanut butter."

I went on shopping, ignoring the insistent voice regarding peanut butter. The voice was annoying, as it continually smacked me—quietly—with its 2x4-sized thought about peanut butter. When I got home after shopping, my son approached me and asked if I got peanut butter, because we were out. I had to laugh, because I ignored the intuitive 2x4 that was trying to get my attention.

Sometimes, the 2x4 can come from people around you. Have you ever been given the suggestion to read a book or watch a show, multiple times from different people, unrelated to each other? Every time this happens, it is the 2x4 getting your attention.

I have had moments when a good friend suggested I read a specific book. When visiting my local coffee shop, I see someone reading this book, and then there is a third 2x4, when someone else suggests this book. The book was not popular or being discussed in mainstream media. There was no reason why all these events happened so close together.

> Explore these 2x4s, because each one leads to something you may need to know or a question that you need answered at that time.

These threads and 2x4s led to a broad overview of what I was dealing with from multiple angles. These areas may never have been explored, unless I was paying attention to these moments or what was being suggested to me. We all have this ability; it is a matter of whether or not we tune in to these moments and trust ourselves to listen.

Chapter 6 Exercise

What Do You Want?

On the surface, we want lots of things, for example, a house, car, money, and security. These things are great. Past the material layer lies respect, love, acceptance, health, joy, happiness, etc. Take your time at this moment to make a list of all of these desires/wants in your life. Divide the list based on external material desires and internal desires that coincide with Who You Are.

Take the time to ask yourself these questions:

- What do I expect of myself?
- What if I achieved my desires, no matter how big?
- What would make me proud of myself?
- What activity am I doing when it feels like time is standing still?
- What brings a sense of security?
- When am I happy or when do I laugh? Who am I with? What am I doing?
- Where do I feel loved and who am I with?
- If I were healthy, what actions would I be doing, and with whom?

Your mind may be racing with more things that you want. Take a look at your list and ask yourself:

> When was the last time you actually asked for these things or made a map of how to get there?

What is Stopping You?

What gets in your way from achieving What You Want? Is it your inner critic? Do you have a moment when you hesitate?

If your actions or thoughts make you feel like you're spinning in a washing machine, *pause them*. It's up to you to make the change.

Is your inner critic stopping you? I began calling my little voice by a name, in order to keep it under control and create more awareness of him. For me, it was a "him," and for you, it could be anyone. This inner critic would help when I needed him, and I would quiet him when I did not want his opinion.

I would also take time being aware of him and loving him. This love was a part of loving myself, honoring the good and bad. I found that if I tried to squash or make my inner critic silent or force him to leave, he only came back stronger. It was not until I listened to this voice that he began to serve me. I did not always take his opinion. In moments when he was being judgmental, I would ask him, "Is this thought true?" It rarely was.

> During your pursuit of What You Want, you may feel like you are bouncing from task to task or idea to idea.

These moments of trying and experimenting are beautiful. But this is when your inner critic wants to have an opinion. If left to his own way, he can become the captain of your thoughts, and he may become a ruthless instrument of judgment. During these moments, *focus* must become your superpower.

In the book, *The Net and the Butterfly: The Art and Practice of Breakthrough Thinking*, the authors Olivia Fox Cabane and Judah Pollack state that we have two sides of our consciousness. The internal voice, the default side, which is the voice of wisdom and intuition that is quiet and is only heard when we are quiet. The other side is where your Ego resides, the loud and sometimes negative voice (your inner critic).

For example, do you ever think of a brilliant solution or idea right as you are going to sleep? This is because the loud Ego voice becomes quiet. You are now listening to your intuition, wisdom, and soul.

The other side of consciousness is your Ego. Your Ego does serve a purpose; it is to remind you of potential dangers and direct your attention to something that may be dangerous. It is when we allow this Ego to overtake our decision-making that it leads to anxiety and stress. This voice tends to dwell on the past, which brings shame and regret, or the voice focuses on the future, which brings anxiety and stress in most cases.

> When we allow this voice to make decisions alone and alter what we want, a challenge may occur. The Ego likes to take the safe route, and it is the first to tell you, "I told you so."

Identify and take time to become intimately aware of both of these voices. Understand who these voices are and what they are telling you. Ask yourself the ultimate question, "Is what my voice tells me true?"

You will be able to tell the difference between both sides, by what these voices say. The quiet voice only speaks in love, gentle reminders, and wise thoughts. The other is loud, judgmental, and tells you of potential dangers.

We are challenged when we are given the label of a disease diagnosis. When we are told we "are" a certain way, we feel as if we have no choice. This feeling of hopelessness or a lack of choice can overtake us, and we are led by fear and the loud, judgmental voice.

Chapter 7

Getting Out of Your Own Way/ Un-Learning the Past/Opening Mindset to Healing

> "Always say 'yes' to the present moment...
> Surrender to what is. Say 'yes' to life – and see how life starts suddenly to start working for you rather than against you."
>
> – Eckhart Tolle, *The Power of Now*

Not Listening to Self & Inner Needs/Inner Voice

During times of fear, we make excuses and justify what we think we need and want. Our fear can leave us with no time, energy, desire, or purpose. The words we tell ourselves (our inner critic) are trying to protect us from the unknown. We are so concerned with failing that we say things like "Don't screw this up," or "I am not good at this," or "Why did I say this?" or "I am such an idiot. How can I be so stupid?"

This negative banter leaves us feeling, acting, and living like we are not enough. We are raised to avoid failure—don't climb on this, watch out for that, be careful. As mentioned in a previous chapter, these scripts, beliefs, and perceived view of the world are developed from the ages of eight to twelve.

When we move into adulthood, we take these perceptions with us and mold them to our adult situations, like being fired, negative family situations, or being diagnosed with a disease. This ingrained fear of failure, mixed with a very real fear of death or a change in Who We Think We Are, leads us to be narrow-minded in our viewpoint.

As we get in our own way, we begin to limit options in order to gain control. This grasping for control can limit us based on our past perceptions and what may have worked or not worked. We stop looking outward and asking for help, and more importantly, we stop looking inward and loving ourselves by slowing down and taking the necessary steps to change our lives for the better. Fear and grasping for control can keep us in our own way and from seeing what is available to us to help us heal.

In 2008, when I paralyzed my leg while shoveling snow, I was blocking my own way and Self. This block, which could not be seen at the time, was as wide and difficult to cross as the Grand Canyon.

The morning I paralyzed my right leg, I woke to a heavy wet Midwestern snow, where each shovelful felt like two hundred pounds. At the time, I was thirty-one, an All-American Triathlete. I felt invincible. I was fit, but I did not work on core strength, besides what was achieved with running, biking, and swimming. I was stressed at work and at home. I tried to mask this with triathlons, endurance events, or anything else that made me feel important.

I noticed at the end of 2007 that my lower back was sore, but as usual, I ignored it. I blamed the increased soreness on training and running the day before. The training must have caught up to me, and I just needed to push through it. I did not give my sore back the attention it needed. I did not give my inner self and the stress I was experiencing the attention it needed. I ignored myself and stopped loving myself for the beautiful soul I was.

I discovered that morning, by not slowing down and listening to my body, my stubborn, egocentric, invincible attitude broke me. So, I continued to lift the heavy snow, which only made my sore back worse. I kept shoveling due to my stubbornness and mental fortitude, thinking that I needed to keep pushing through the pain. For some reason, I thought I needed to finish the job.

I remember pushing the shovel into the snow, collecting as much wet cold mess as I could, planting my feet, and attempting to throw it. As the snow left the shovel, I felt the pain in my back grow to an obvious injury. I fell to my knees. Something was wrong, and as I stood up; I noticed my right leg did not work as it should. I tried to ignore the injury but knew something was seriously wrong. The injury was tough to ignore, due to the extreme amount of pain. I also noticed I could not raise myself on my right toes, and my right foot would drop and drag when I walked.

The pain remained after the shoveling accident and did not improve after a few days. Fear started to set in. I was scared and angry, and I avoided seeing doctors because I did not want to realize that it could be much worse. I was in denial and thought I just needed to work through the pain. I could no longer sit in meetings, drive my car, or stand for long periods without extreme pain. Once it was affecting my daily life, I could not ignore it any further.

Soon after this realization, my first step was to call the chiropractor's office I had visited while racing, to ask their opinion and schedule an appointment. One of these chiropractors was Paul, a friend who was finishing his degree at a local large chiropractic school. Instead of adjusting me, he took his time helping me relieve the pain by using active release therapy (ART). After Paul got me pain-free after a few treatments, my focus changed to getting my right leg to work so I could run again. Paul knew and understood that I wanted to avoid surgery, due to the horror stories I heard from others who had undergone back surgery. In hindsight, I made some terrible decisions out of fear; they are still costing me.

I managed to get in my own way, and my view became narrow, only focused on one method of treatment. I was no longer listening to anyone, even myself. I knew what I wanted, and at the time, I believed I knew who I was. As I look back now, I was scared and ignorant, and I make this statement with love.

My views at the time of who I was and what I wanted were non-negotiable, not up for interpretation. I became so focused on the material and Ego of what I wanted that I forgot to think about and love me. The more I focused on the material, outside reality and my accomplishments, the harder it became to listen. The noise of fear and my Ego, which reminded me that I screwed up, drowned out the most important voice I needed to hear: My Self-love.

I was having a surface-level conversation with myself and those around me. I was afraid to go deeper and face the reality of what was going on. I continued to bury my head in the sand, hoping the problems would magically go away.

Fear & Physiology & Excuses

It is easy, in the moment of fear, to avoid yourself and the reality of what is happening.

We operate with animal instincts when under fear. Imagine the last time you were angry: Did you say the most brilliant remarks that caused the individual to ponder and stop in their tracks? No, you most likely did not. If you did, can you justify the reaction and what you said?

Human beings, who are animals when under stress or in fear, have an area of the brain that controls these emotional reactions: the amygdala.

The amygdala is a small, almond-shaped cluster in the center of the brain. It is our fight, flight, or freeze override. This part of our brain is the source of our automatic responses, trying to keep us out of danger and alive.

Imagine it is 7,000 years ago, and you exit your shelter to find a bear standing in front of you. What do you do? Try to talk to the bear and reason with it? See if it wants to be petted? Try to ride it to your friend's shelter? No, you either run, defend yourself, or freeze when seeing the bear. If you did not react in a split second to this dangerous situation, you could be lunch.

In today's world, I hope you do not encounter a bear when leaving the house, but you may encounter someone slamming their brakes unexpectedly in front of you on your drive to work.

Did you think about slamming on your brakes, or did you immediately hit the brakes with no thought? At the time it happens, you may feel your heart race, your hands become cold or sweaty. Or you may say something that you are not proud of. All of this is your brain's attempt to keep you safe and alive.

When your amygdala takes over, two chemicals are released: adrenaline (aka, epinephrine) and cortisol, which is known as the stress hormone.

Adrenaline causes you to run faster and become stronger, and cortisol affects clarity of thought, so you follow the fight, flight, or freeze response, without thinking. In fact, the nerves from your eyes and ears do not pass through the logic center of your brain, your prefrontal cortex; instead, these nerves are directly wired to your amygdala.

Your fight-or-flight center controls your first reactionary choice when you encounter danger. If your amygdala senses danger, even in a minor amount, adrenaline is immediately released, and cortisol quickly follows. This adrenaline response can even happen under a minor amount of fear or stress.

But how do we know how to react if the logic center of our brains has been turned off by cortisol? The automatic decision of how to respond or what to do comes from another area in the brain called the basal ganglia, where long-term memory and thoughts are stored. Your Basal Ganglia receives its information from activities you have practiced over and over, like hitting the brake in your car in a moment of danger.

What have you practiced over and over so much that you can do it in your sleep? This will be what your amygdala accesses to make its choice to keep you alive.

When we are diagnosed with a disease and faced with our own mortality, we may begin developing the mindset that we are going to be sick or maybe even die. We begin to develop and store this new thought in our Basal Ganglia. You stop listening to others because of fear, or you make the statement to others: "You have no idea how I feel."

You may continue to put up your walls and push others away. The fear of losing who you Believe you are, and maybe even your own life, may have you listening to one viewpoint, keeping you from exploring other options. It's like putting on headphones and the only words you hear are the ones you want to hear.

What sometimes challenges our perceived choices is the fear, stress, and loss of our past selves. The cascading spiral downward leads to an increased response from our amygdala and more cortisol. What if you were aware of the fear and limiting response, and instead, remained open to possibility, no matter what? What if your identity was one that was serving you instead of limiting you?

Making Choices Out of Fear

Viewing a diagnosis through the lens of fear makes you feel like you have no other options. This scenario that I described is one that I have felt throughout my life and is very real. The fear of our own lives being changed or ending can begin to get in our own way. We can adopt a limiting perspective based on how we feel. These feelings can be terrible and leave us without movement, bodily functions, or hope. Those around us want to help us any way they can, but they can feel as lost as we are.

God, Universe, Source, or whatever you believe, has a great way of giving you the answer and providing guides for healing, but the teacher and healer can only appear when the student is ready. If I would have gotten out of my own way and begun listening, I may have made different decisions earlier or asked different questions that led me to answers sooner. As I spoke with Paul and other doctors, I was being told that timing was important with any motor control issue.

All I heard was *blah, blah, blah*. I told myself that I was tough and an All-American Triathlete. That was my "identity" at that time. I was in my own way, and whether I thought I could or could not, I was right.

What if your life has just been turned upside down by a diagnosis? The fear, anger, shame, or sense of loss from the diagnosis may keep you frozen or have you making a choice out of this fear.

If you have ever experienced a diagnosis delivered by a doctor, you may only do what the doctor says, out of fear. Your response may be to take the doctor's advice immediately as the only option, but does this choice align with What You Want and Who You Are, your *Identity* and *Belief of Self*?

Often, we do not want to be defined in terms of a medical label and have our humanity reduced to a diagnosis, so we may flee in denial from our diagnosis. What were you telling yourself before the doctor's appointment? Was your mindset one of possibility and a search for options?

These thoughts of possibility and ability to slow down stem from your identity. For example, if I identify myself as an Ironman, able to swim, bike, and run long distances in one day, then competing and finishing the race seems possible. If I am told and believe I cannot do it, I immediately question why I am undertaking this endeavor, which may lead me to not finish the race.

When we are diagnosed with a disease, it is not always out of the blue. We usually notice symptoms. These symptoms cause us to go to the doctor, and possibly research our symptoms on WebMD, which is not always encouraging and sometimes tells us that our hangnail could be cancer.

I would like to offer a quick disclaimer regarding using the internet to diagnose:

Of course, we've all looked up our symptoms and self-diagnosed. But it's important to remember that, unless you have a medical degree and lab tests have been done, you don't really know what your symptoms indicate. Don't get discouraged by anything you read on the internet. Try to use that information to prepare yourself, then go in and describe the symptoms to your doctor. Let the medical professionals conduct the right tests and leave the diagnoses up to them. If you have further questions or want a second opinion, you're within your rights to seek additional information afterward. But, please, if you're experiencing symptoms, get them checked out by a licensed, practicing medical professional.

The fear of the unknown is built before you go into the doctor's office. The one thing we do not address is the identity and Belief of Who We Are and What We Want. Having a plan based on your self-perceived identity before you step foot in the doctor's office, or even if you have already been and started to walk down the road, it is never too late to establish your identity. Your identity grounds you, and the statement usually starts with *I am*.

Is This True?

My choice to overcome my paralyzed leg and start racing again became a primary thought and desire. When the negative voice became loud, as discussed in Chapter 6, I would remind myself of the story of Rick and Dick Hoyt. These two extraordinary individuals went on to become Team Hoyt.

Team Hoyt is made up of father and son, Richard "Dick" Hoyt (born June 1, 1940) and Richard "Rick" Hoyt, Jr. (born January 10, 1962). They have competed together in various athletic endeavors, including marathons and multiple Ironman Triathlons. I was always inspired because Rick has cerebral palsy. During their competitions, Dick pulls Rick in a special boat as they swim, carries Rick in a special seat on the front of the bicycle, and pushes him in a special wheelchair jogger during the marathon. They have finished every Ironman they competed in, and every time Rick and Dick crossed the finish line with joy, smiles light up the stands. You can see awe and tears on the faces of all the fans witnessing the moment.

These acts of self-encouragement and building my mental muscle were as important as building my aerobic capacity to handle the long day of work that lay ahead of me. At this time, I had friends who had completed Ironman and mentioned the mental struggle during the race.

I approached Ironman like I did all the other races I had completed. Work hard enough, so there was no doubt or fear. What was I accomplishing with working hard beyond my perceived ability? Was I changing my mindset, one pedal stroke and foot strike at a time?

> *Mindset* is defined as the established set of attitudes held by someone.

My attitude at the beginning of training was not positive, and the frustration of having my leg still collapse when stepping up on a curb did not help.

So, I made a conscious effort to approach what I thought about myself and what I told myself. Being aware of the negative internal banter, thinking about my past or slumping into victimhood, allowed me to make a different choice. When the inner critic would start, I would say, "Stop." Sometimes, I physically stopped.

Once the voice stopped and I had its attention, I would ask the voice, "Is this true?"

The voice could never answer this question, because in each case, it was wrong. At the time, I viewed mindset as two separate aspects of thought—the old way and the new way. The old way involved "should have," blame, victimization, anger, and depression. The new way included encouragement, support, and love for me.

This way of thinking about mindset got me in trouble. I found myself with an attitude of right and wrong. The little voice had something to point out every time it was not at a place where I believed was right. This way of thinking about things in terms of polar opposites—right or wrong—was not healthy. The thought pattern I was trying to adjust was already stacked against me, with 70-80 percent of my thoughts being negative.

It was like going to all-day meetings with a bad cold, always being reminded that you are still sick. I was making the mental part of the journey, which required no physical effort, exhausting. Why couldn't all my thoughts, no matter what they were, just be that—a thought, and nothing more? Why did it have to be *right* or *wrong*? The thoughts were only thoughts.

A New Voice

As I explored this concept of the weight of my thoughts and why I gave some more credit than others, I started to notice another voice rise up. This voice provided encouragement, even though it was very quiet, and I had to listen fully to hear it. Over time, I slowly began to change and made this mental flip. This change in how

I approached my thoughts began to take the pressure off. It needed time, and I used training for Ironman to give it the time it needed.

If you asked me in December of 2010, the month after I signed up for Ironman, if I could swim 2.4 miles, bike another 112 miles, and then run a marathon of 26.2 miles, I would have laughed. I knew it was going to take a year of slowly progressing forward with a specific, intentional plan. Instead of my attitude and thoughts being an overnight transition, they became a slow, methodical progression.

I knew that if I was going to succeed, it would take time. This is true whether we're talking about a competition, a new job, or adjusting to a major life change, such as a new child or disease diagnosis. I knew I would have to build up my strength and endurance, and I remind you that you, too, will need to build up strength and endurance.

Developing a new voice helped me, and it could help you too. Here's what my new voice sounded like. I knew it was my new voice when it was loving, kind, graceful, and encouraging, no matter what it said. I began to approach my mindset like training for Ironman. Along with building my strength and endurance, I was going to build my mental muscle. At times when I was struggling, down on myself, or not performing the way I wanted, I automatically went to my new healthy mindset of what I wanted with encouraging love, rather than an old, limiting thought pattern.

Becoming A Master/New Voice Starts with New Thoughts

Malcolm Gladwell in his book *Outliers* claims that in order to become a master at anything, it takes 10,000 hours. To become a master at anything, it involves practice.

For example, if you desire to become a concert pianist, it will take possibly 10,000 hours of practice until the music flows through you. When you start the journey, it may have seemed clumsy, and you found yourself looking at your hands with intense concentration. Then, through practice and time, it became a more automatic thought process, an ingrained neural pathway.

The pathways along which information travels through the neurons (nerve cells) of the brain can be compared with the paths through a forest. Every time you learn something, neural circuits are altered in your brain. When we engage in a thought or exercise less frequently, it is like walking through the woods—there is no clear path. You may stumble or possibly feel like you're lost. The neural pathway has not begun wiring together yet.

> When we engage more often in the thoughts or practiced activity, we gain Awareness as it becomes easier. There still may be times when you stumble, you may still have questions, but they become less frequent. The wiring of the pathway begins to connect.

As we practice more and more, you find it becoming more automatic and easier. You may feel more joy, confidence, and belief in your ability. Your thoughts follow, with words like "Keep trying. That was fun." Any words of encouragement. This encouragement leads to more practice and the task or thought that seemed difficult or impossible at the beginning now feels automatic. You may have noticed your identity shift to what you wanted, and you are no longer thinking about how difficult it is. You may start to think in terms of joy and Belief. Life may feel easier, but it would not have begun to be this way, unless you took the first step and decided to make a change.

As human beings, we survive and thrive by having automatic thoughts to situations or events. For example, stop and remember the last time you went into a department store where you were asked, "Can I help you?" and you responded, "No," or some version of it. That is your automatic neural pathway in action. You may have not even thought of this statement; it just rolled out of your mouth.

> If 70–80 percent of our thoughts every day
> are negative, that is a lot of practice,
> in the direction we do not want.

If you continually practice negative thoughts, are you not developing this muscle, like the concert pianist? You may realize that you have become a master of your negative thoughts, clouding your self-love. You may feel as if you are in the rut of your negative automatic neural thought pathway. Can you imagine how automatic and engrained most of our thoughts are? Think about your common responses or thoughts to situations throughout your day. These automatic thoughts begin to shape your beliefs, moods, behavior, and actions.

The last thing I wanted was the task of monitoring every thought, but I knew it was critical to find a way out of the dangerous thoughts I was regularly thinking. I approached my thoughts and attitude like training for Ironman. It was going to take a little at a time, until it was conducted effortlessly. I prepared for the uncoordinated, wobbly moments in my thoughts, like riding my bike for a few hours and then running right after.

Yes, it is exhausting and frustrating to catch yourself every time the negative thoughts creep in and you realize you have been thinking about them for a while, but I had a plan. I treated changing my mindset like a series of steps. I began by making a list of regular, recurring, automatic thoughts, just to be aware of them. As I became aware of these thoughts, I started to see the triggers or situations that led to the negative thoughts.

For example, If I started to become discouraged and down on myself, I might catch myself thinking, "There is no way I am going to complete this monumental task." Once I realized what I was thinking, I stopped and looked at what happened before the thought. Was I training too hard? Was I stressed out at work? Had I just gotten in an argument with a loved one? Now that I was aware of the thoughts and realized that it was just a thought, I began to reframe it.

I began to attach new thoughts to these situations. I attached a thought of encouragement I wanted, not one of victimhood or excuses. I began to make a mental list and sometimes wrote down the positive thoughts and mantras I wanted to adopt. I even went as far as taping some of these thoughts to the top bar of my bicycle, so I was forced to stare at them when I trained. I began to think of the response I wanted to have to these situations and how I wanted to be. Then I practiced, like the concert pianist. If I felt the negative voice creeping in, which it often did, I would give it love, thank it, and then make it go sit on the curb.

Once I stopped mentally punishing myself for every thought I was trying to avoid and reframed the thought, I noticed my belief change. Then my behavior changed, and I stopped being so critical and judgmental of myself. The more I practiced, the easier it was to identify the trigger events before they happened. The ability to continually produce the responses I wanted automatically were easier when I knew the trigger events.

It's like how they tell you in driver's education classes not to look only twenty feet in front of the car you're driving, but to look two hundred yards ahead, so you can anticipate danger in different situations. After time and practice, thinking this way became automatic.

As I look back now, I began to understand that who I thought I was, and my mindset allowed Belief to grow. I sowed a seed of Belief and watered it with behavior and energy as it grew into a tree, matching who I believed I was.

Opening up to Others' Ways

After I paralyzed my leg, it was not until the fourth month after the injury that I started to pay attention and listen to what others were saying. I had lost 90 percent of my muscle mass out of my right leg, and my chiropractor-friend Paul had a difficult conversation with me. He explained that if I did not do something else, I would lose full functionality of the right leg. Losing this functionality would lead to the choice of amputation.

I humbly started paying attention and began looking at other options. All I could think about was not being able to run again, which I missed. I also missed my bike and the long meditative rides it gave. My singular identity and view of Who I Thought I Was did not exist anymore. I was too scared to slow down, listen, and accept what had happened. I was getting in my own way, and I could not see it. Looking back at the stress during this time, mixed with my stubbornness, kept me from seeing that I was enough, and it was okay to make a mistake and slow down. I was not looking for, or aware of, another step, I did not know what to do, and I slipped into victimhood as the fear grew. I was running from my own healing and those around me who wanted to help.

It is apparent, now, what I was thinking and feeling; it is apparent why I made the choices I made, creating my current reality. I was lost, and I felt like I lost 90 percent of my self-worth along with my leg. I felt my worth was wrapped up in physical activity, awards, and my ego of winning races. When my identity was stripped, I did not know who I was, or what I wanted. The feeling of not being good enough was always in my subconscious mind. I did not take the time to understand and avoided these two very important questions at a deeper level for many years after this life-changing injury.

> My predominant negative thought pattern became practiced and ingrained into the beliefs of Who I Thought I Was. Rising out of the state I was in was going to take surrendering and slowing down enough to listen.

New Medical Perspectives

As I began to listen about other options to help my leg, a good friend suggested a neurologist who specialized in back injuries. I did not hesitate and made an appointment with the neurologist. After the doctor reviewed my MRI at our appointment, he suggested surgery and presented the option of a microlaminectomy. During the microlaminectomy procedure, he would insert a tube the width of an index finger into my lower spine. The tube would allow him to insert instruments to clean the scar tissue and blown disc from the nerves that blocked the messages to my right leg and foot. It seemed like the least invasive option, but it came with a catch. During the procedure, he would be working close to other areas important for lower-limb functionality. If there was a slip and other areas were damaged, he could paralyze me from the waist down. He offered me a 50 percent chance of the procedure working.

Time was of the essence, and knew I only had a few days to make this decision. I had to rely on others and trust them, so I said, "Yes. Let's go ahead with the surgery." At this time, I asked myself, "Why am I better, more knowledgeable, or wiser than the doctor? He went to med school."

My lack of self-worth and thinking that I was smart enough kept me from typing my injury into a Google search to see what other options were available. I stopped being curious, and the fear of not running or competing again kept me from getting out of my own way, trusting my intuition, and slowing down enough to listen.

I was fortunate that I met the right doctor, and the procedure was successful. I walked out of the surgery center and was looking at a three-year rehabilitation of my right leg.

Make Every Day a 'Hell Yes' Day

When was the last time you went left when everyone else went right? In the end, it may not have gone as planned, but it took your life in an unintended direction. As I continued to study, I made choices because I wanted to, not because I had to. Also, it became natural to follow the paths that left me feeling better.

> You are given a choice, every single day.
> In some cases, a multitude of these choices
> can happen, all within a matter of minutes.
> We filter our choices through
> Who You Think You Are and What You Want.

For example, for the health of my marriage, I had to make a choice on where I spend my time. I remember the time when my son was newly born, and I was training for the triathlon, a lot. This involved very early mornings, and most

Saturdays I was not home for my then-wife and our new son. When asked if I wanted to golf on Sunday, the answer was always "No." I had to make a choice on what I wanted, and my priorities were focused on my home and racing. I read an article from Derek Sivers from his book *Anything You Want,* in which he makes the statement, "If it is not a 'hell yeah,' then it is a 'no.'"

We are the ones who have to be okay with the choices we make. What is difficult is when there is not a good choice either way. Making a decision can be gut wrenching and leave us feeling frozen, so we do not make any choice. Our fear sometimes freezes us in indecision, and our minds race with possibilities and "what if" scenarios. We cascade through these scenarios, leaving us frozen.

What if I make the wrong decision? What if this decision leaves me feeling worse?

Have you ever sat and thought about how that *feels* inside your body? We often let our executive function, our brains, determine our fate, and we discredit or stop listening to anything else, even ourselves.

This executive function is not always accurate. Have you ever made a bad decision while your body or "gut" was telling you "No"?

Chapter 7 Exercise

Talking Back to Inner Voice

This exercise is not meant to put you in guilt, shame or make you feel bad about yourself.

Your first step is to become aware of your thoughts, good or bad.

In your journal, draw a line down the center of a page to divide the page in half. For five minutes, sit and think about the thoughts you regularly have about yourself and categorize them appropriately:

On the *left* column, write your *negative* thoughts.

Along the *right* column, write your *positive* thoughts.

Now, fold up this journal page and put it in your pocket (or purse, backpack, or other easily accessible area you will have with you all day).

As you go about your day, make notes of the thoughts you have.

If the judgmental voice starts to creep in your head and says negative things that make you feel small and limited, breathe through those moments. Let them pass. You are just observing, like a scientist.

After a day or two of adding to your list, you will have a pretty thorough list.

Then, find a quiet space and cover the right side of the page so you can address the negative thoughts on the list. Ask this question for each:

"Is this true?"

Think about your answer. Be honest with yourself.

Don't let the judgmental voice in your head answer for you, even though it will try.

This question will be the *only one* that your internal critic and negative voice cannot answer, because really, what that voice says is not true. It is a limited perception of the situation. Like I tell my kids: There are three sides to a story – yours, theirs, and the *truth*.

Conclusion

Try not to not dwell in the past, learn from it. Understand the triggers and moments that led you here. The past can lead to shame, regret, and a case of the "should'ves."

I should have done this. I shouldn't have done that.

> We cannot change the past;
> we can only learn from it.

What was your mindset in the months and years leading to the diagnosis you received? Were you stressed? On medication? Injured? Exposed to toxins in your food and environment?

Some of the time, it is not only one of these but a mixture of multiple factors. The only way you can avoid the pothole on the road is to know where it is.

Take time to look inward with no judgment. This is not the time to put blame on anyone or anything; it is time to learn and heal.

> You can heal.
> A diagnosis is an opportunity for
> you to slow down and discover
> the root cause within yourself.

Remember, whether you think you can or think you cannot, you're right!

You have the power and means to educate yourself, no matter how much money you have or don't have. Nothing is stopping you but you. In the least, I hope you make the choice to become curious and begin exploring for your own sake.

Be the leader, CEO, and champion of your health. Build a team that supports your choices, encouraging you along your path. Above all, slow down and love yourself, because you are enough and worth every second.

Chapter 8

Mindset to Heal

"Keep your thoughts positive because your thoughts become your words. Keep your words positive because your words become your behavior. Keep your behavior positive because your behavior becomes your habits. Keep your habits positive because your habits become your values. Keep your values positive because your values become your destiny."

– Mahatma Gandhi, *Open Your Mind, Open Your Life*

On a cold fall day during a long training run, I could feel the crisp air on my cheeks and see the early morning frost on the grass before the sun had its way of evaporating the reminder of winter coming. As I ran down a rarely used paved farm road, I could smell the peaceful fall air and the drying corn in the farm's field next to me, calling out to be harvested.

I saw, up ahead, a flock of blackbirds pouring out of a tight valley, maybe fifty feet wide. I could hear the flutter of a thousand wings, as I witnessed a dance in perfect form and harmony. I continued to run toward the sound, and when I was about twenty yards away, I could see a flock of more than one hundred birds leave the valley and enter a large dense tree on the edge of the road. As one flock flew into the tree, another flock of more than one hundred birds, which I could not see, left the large tree and poured into the large field filled with the drying corn, about one hundred yards away.

As I stood there in awe of the dance, I felt an intense peace wash over me, witness to the flow of life. The birds did not stop or slow the dance. They trusted me, standing there, just as each group trusted the group before them.

For twenty minutes, I stood there and began thinking about the harmony of life. No will was being forced upon this dance. No director ensured the perfect timing. It was trust and Belief in motion.

> When I am feeling frustrated or overwhelmed by life, I think back to this moment and realize that God, Universe, Source does all of the flow of life in perfect timing.

When I think about all the negative moments and the reasons I give myself about why "it will not work," I am reminded of all the ways it *will* work. This brings me hope and the reminder that we are all meant for the highest and best of life, no matter the situation. We must step out of the way of trying to direct the flow; we must trust that everything in front of us is a transition, from the forest of the unknown to an open field of possibility.

Mind Over Matter

As I clicked the button to submit my registration and commitment to Ironman Arizona, I felt a wave of nausea creep over me. At the time, I had bankrupted my company, and I was two years into a three-year process of gaining strength and functionality back to the right leg I had paralyzed two years earlier. I knew the steps I needed to take to train for such a long endurance event, as I had competed in over one hundred triathlons before my injury. The challenge was going to be to continue training, even though I could not raise and support myself on my right toes. I knew what I wanted—to complete a journey I had started years before and be an Ironman.

My leg was starting to come back, but it was not the same. My running was labored, biking was not even close to where it was, and swimming was arduous. The little voice in my head was not my friend. I was tired of being reminded why signing up for Ironman was a bad idea.

My attitude and mental state would be considered severe depression, at best. In addition to the paralysis, I had put my family in debt and had no income. Thoughts of suicide plagued me. For my own mental well-being and safety, I knew I needed to change this depressed thought pattern, and I was relying on Ironman to mask my pain. Based on my experience of being a competitive triathlete, I knew Ironman was 75 percent mental, and I was going to have a lot of time alone to process what happened. I had a year to train for the epic event, and something had to change. Either my leg would start working again, or maybe, I could find myself again.

I started building the mental muscle of thinking and believing that I could reach this goal. I needed to get out of the dark hole I had constructed for myself. I used the long training rides, followed by long training runs, as mental therapy.

A small ember of Belief began to grow, and I felt myself encouraged to train. I wanted my old life of being an athlete back, and being dubbed an "Ironman" had a nice ring to it. I was willing to do the work because that is what I wanted.

The first step was to fan the flames of Belief and ignore negative thoughts. My journey not only involved training my body to finish Ironman but also training my mind into a strong belief of knowing that I could. My inner voice was always a challenge, and at times, he crept up so quietly and slyly that I remember thinking the negative thoughts, as if they were always there.

I wanted to get control of this voice, to make it shut up. I tried driving the voice to exhaustion, yelling at it, numbing it with alcohol, anything to get it to stop talking. I read countless books and started to attend church again to distract the insistent negative voice.

I had not started meditating yet. (I didn't even know how!) Out of frustration one day, while out on my bike, I started paying close attention to the voice, instead of constantly trying to quiet it. As I listened to it, without always believing it, the voice became quieter.

Motivational Stories

During this time, I also used motivational stories of people who achieved the impossible, especially when the negative voice became too loud. One story in particular that I loved was the story of Rick and Dick Hoyt, who were mentioned earlier.

I was also inspired by stories of Sarah Reinertsen. In 2005, Reinertsen became the first female leg amputee to ever finish Ironman in Kona, Hawaii. I remember meeting Sarah when earning my All-American Triathlete designation at the half-Ironman distance (1.2-mile swim, 56-mile bike, 13.1-mile run) during the Chicago Triathlon. As we fired up a conversation before the race, I would never have imagined that her story would help me complete my Ironman after my own injuries.

I was also inspired by the story of Lance Armstrong. Say what you wish about Lance, he inspired a movement of possibility in so many cyclists. While training during his multiple Tour de France wins, Armstrong was reported to say, "You can quit and no one will care, but you will always know."

I taped this quote to the top tube of my bicycle and stared at it when I became discouraged during the long, lonely training rides. These stories became a bedrock for me, on which to find the positive lessons life offered. When I felt the negative voice creep in, I quieted it by reminding myself: Things could be much worse. If those individuals rose above those moments, so could I.

My only limitation became me. I was limited only by whether I believed and knew that I would cross the finish line on November 20, 2011.

Time Is Important/Sense of Urgency

During this life-changing event, I learned, over time, that it is critical to slow down and listen. We can be blind to the realization that we are, in our own ways, making our situation worse. We never know when a life-changing decision or event may be given to us. During these moments, sometimes the best (and possibly only) avenue and choice we can make is to stop and go inside ourselves. Taking time for yourself can be critical, and often, a deep breath, or sitting quietly in meditation or prayer, or a walk alone, listening, can be the most important step you take.

As I sat quietly, reflecting on my life and the events that led me to the point of writing this book, questions arose that guided me to continue through the storm of life. These questions were humbling and led to a great deal of thought and introspection. Some of the questions came from mentors, others came from within and a higher knowing, while others came when I least expected them. If I had not slowed down and been open to hearing these moments, I would have missed them.

We will reflect on these questions later in the chapter, but let's explore the reasons for them. These questions are meant to make you take a step back, slow down, and look inside yourself for the answers beckoning to be released. *You* are the reason and solution for your healing, no one else.

A pill or treatment is meant to fix the symptom, and in some cases, can cure your issue, but in other cases, it cannot. If you are healed by taking the pill or injection, that is great! The issue with a quick fix is that it allows you to avoid the major reason that the diagnosis or disease may have come to be.

> This mask of the "quick fix" may keep you from addressing what is truly important: You.

I had to come to the realization in my life that I am in control of anything and everything that happens to me. In the book *Right Now* by Steve Chandler, he describes the concept of cause and explains that *we*, each of us, are the cause. This might be difficult to hear, especially with what you are experiencing and going through. Let's slow down a little and explore the concept Steve is describing.

Your viewpoints, actions, beliefs, opinions, and responses are based on your perceptions of events. When my kids were arguing over a situation or event and were trying to explain to me who was at fault, I told them, "There are three sides to this story—yours, theirs, and the truth."

Once you realize that you are the cause of all events in your life – good or bad – you can take ownership, without bringing guilt, shame, or playing the victim. Instead, your ownership will come from a place of healing and responsibility. If you caused the event, then you can cause the outcome you want in any situation or event.

If my leg was paralyzed because I decided not to work on my core strength—ignoring my sore back, allowing anger and stress to dictate my actions, going out that morning to shovel snow in frustration—maybe I would not be where I am today. Instead of "shoulding" all over myself, I can go inward, realizing that I was the cause. Then, I make the decision to be the cause of what I want my life to be after this life-changing event.

When I first heard this statement, my Ego did not agree with the author. No, I would not cause an injury of this magnitude for myself intentionally, but deep down, I knew Chandler was right. As I dissected how this injury came to be, I could point back to and learn from the many choices I made leading up to it. I was choosing to learn from my experiences, because that is all we can do with the past.

> Take the time to learn from the past
> and address why it happened that way.

The Importance of Breath

As you read this chapter, you may be thinking about your own journey and responsibility you have to your life, up to this moment. You may feel stuck, frustrated, or even angry, and that is all okay. You may begin to realize that you have the choice to feel this way or not, and you may decide that you do not want to feel negative emotions but emotions of joy and love, instead.

Belief to Heal

> If you are feeling stuck, stop and ask yourself:
> *Which way feels good?*

The negative emotion or what you tell yourself is a guidepost, a moment of Awareness, as discussed in earlier chapters. It is our opportunity to create the life that we want, and that all begins with slowing down and focusing on the simple act of breathing.

In the time it took you to read these last few sentences, you have taken three or four breaths. When you are in a moment of feeling stuck, not able to make a decision due to avoidance, or if no good choice is in front of you—breathe. Let's begin right now by taking five deep breaths.

> Start by sitting quietly in a safe place.
> Close your eyes.
> Ground your feet to the floor, and imagine your feet are growing roots into the earth.

Take a long deep breath in through your nose, and blow it out through your mouth, slowly and deliberately. Continue this breath four more times, imagining the roots of your feet grounding to earth and a beautiful light resonating from your heart.

As you breathe in, imagine each deep breath filling your heart center. As you complete your fifth breath, slowly begin to open your eyes, and enter back into the space you are in.

> How do you feel?

We go through life so fast, solving problems and searching for the perfect answer. When we move too quickly, we forget to slow down and use the other side of our consciousness. The side of our consciousness, which is not affected by the hormones and chemicals that are created by fear. During a time when we experience fear, we release adrenaline that helps us fight, flee, or freeze in a situation, as discussed in earlier chapters.

As you know, this response also blocks clarity of thought and our ability to listen. When we take a few deep breaths through fearful moments, we begin to listen and hear the ever-present voice inside our minds. When we slow down and breathe during these moments of fear, we can also hear a quieter voice coming from Source, Universe, God, or whatever higher power you believe in.

> You will find that this voice *loves* you
> and is going to lead you down another path,
> one step at a time.

When you let the side of your consciousness not affected by fear become involved, you will see the situation from a different angle. During this time, curiosity or questions may arise. Explore these questions and follow the threads of curiosity. With any diagnosis, we have time to slow ourselves, even if it is only for a few moments.

> Always remember during this time:
> There is no right or wrong. There just *is*.

You are the master of your domain, and it is your choice how you respond and live. Living in today's day and age we are blessed to have mass amounts of information at our fingertips very quickly.

Become curious about the choices that lie in front of you. Take time to slow down, read, or ask questions. Go to seminars. Seek out teachers, gurus, and guides. Become aware of what is around you. Breathe and listen to the quiet moments of your life that are trying to get your attention. The loud moments and voices are driven by fear and your Ego, trying to keep you safe. The voice in your head which is based in Love, our ultimate guide from Source, is quiet; sometimes, it can be muted and go unnoticed.

Do Your Own Research

Today, we are made to believe that there is only one way. When you make a choice, what is the harm in knowing as much as you can? During this journey, my diagnosis became the best gift ever handed to me, because I woke up and started to pay attention to something bigger than myself.

The choice that I made and Believe in was not immediate. I made the choice to control MS using unconventional means. I began using food as medicine and by eliminating toxins from my food and environment. I practice meditation and set boundaries to reduce stress. I also exercise to remain fit and active, and I use acupuncture along with other therapeutic means that help me feel better daily.

What has worked for me may not correlate to you, as we are all different. I encourage you to seek your own teachers, guides, doctors, and modalities that help you feel better.

This journey is not a one-size-fits-all situation. It is a journey of knowing yourself at a deeper level, which involves love and patience. I am continuing to remain curious about my choice, and I peel back the layers of the proverbial onion daily.

This journey required me to pay close attention to what I eat and how I feel. I first started my journey of addressing MS by reading *Medical Medium* by Anthony William. This book led me to reduce daily toxins and heavy metals in my diet.

As I explored additional steps, I came to Dr. Terry Wahls' research on how to reduce inflammation. These are two of many steps you may take, and you will discover others that help your symptoms. Through this journey, I discovered that this is a path I will happily be on, for the rest of my life.

I researched various means that have healed others, and the reasons why those means work, I decided to alter my diet. I avoid glyphosate (Roundup), which is spread on many growing grains. I avoid foods that have been genetically modified and those that are exposed to toxins, such as corn, soy, dairy, gluten, pork, or eggs. It may seem severe, but I notice that when I eat these items, I have a negative reaction. Sometimes, it's a slight reaction and sometimes it's severe, but all the time, I want to avoid it.

I made my choice and have my reasons, based on what I wanted and how I feel. After making these choices, I sometimes come upon those who have a comment about my choices, including my family and friends. Yes, it can make it harder and seed doubt, but it also gives me resolve to continue my education and practices.

> In the end, other people
> do not have to live your life.
> You do.

Out of all the research conducted, certifications gained, and doctors spoken to, I learned that these options seemed best for me. I continue to feel good, as I make this choice for me. I have created milestones and goals based on activity and general well-being. I created a plan, which involved a daily dose of self-love and patience.

Even as I have overcome my symptoms and reversed MS, I do not see myself changing anytime soon. My health and mood have improved, and I am meeting the milestones I set forth. At times, yes, I still have moments when I do not feel my best, but I quickly correlate them to what I eat, what activities I am performing, and my stress levels.

During this journey, I have become a certified health coach, written this book, and spoken on the TEDx stage. I began to see the blessings, lessons, and opportunities that life has to offer. It was all there before my MS diagnosis, but I was focused on my external world so much that I did not listen to the joy.

Your choice is yours, and as my daughter says, "You do you." And you have your reasons. This does not mean that once a choice is made, all others go away. I want to challenge you to become a master at knowing and understanding where you are going and why.

I remember talking to my doctor, who asked me what I was doing and how. As I explained my protocol, she could not confirm or deny the path I was on as a right or wrong one. When I talked to her about nutrition and food as a mode of healing, she was more curious than probing. The looks she gave and the small-but-noticeable doubt she had could have led into and built upon any doubt I had and my choices. It was important at the time that my choice was open to listen to the awareness of myself, and how I was feeling, but also the conviction to remain on the path I chose.

Whatever choice you make and the threads you follow, it is your choice. Be confident in knowing that you are taking your health into your own hands and that you are looking at every angle. It is your health, your life, your story, and no one can live this life for you. You have to wake up every morning and deal with the little voice that no one but you can hear. You have a choice of what the little voice says and how it makes you feel. You have a choice to become aware of the little voice in your mind, and what is around you as your intuition tries to get your attention.

Chapter 8 Exercise
Ask Yourself the Following Questions

As I healed and started to feel better, I was led toward some important questions that had me explore deep within my soul and my reasons for healing. Although these questions could have been difficult or easy to answer, they had me exploring possible causes of stress and fear that I was trying to avoid or cover up. As I explored these questions, my awareness of what was important to me grew, along with the triggers that kept me in Fear.

For the next exercise, I would like you to sit with your journal and ask yourself these questions:

- What am I choosing to ignore and pretend not to understand?
- How is this diagnosis or event currently impacting me?
- What am I avoiding?
- What am I afraid of?
- What am I being told that does not feel right?
- What have I not been listening or paying attention to?
- What do I not want?

Write down your answers in your journal and reflect on your answers when you feel out of balance or critical of your choices.

Conclusion

You have the opportunity to be the master of your domain. Taking control of your thoughts takes practice, along with intention and desire to want a different outcome. I remember explaining and working with a client through these steps. During our second coaching session, the client told me that these steps were not working, that they were still having thoughts that made them feel terrible. Those perceived terrible thoughts led the individual to the choices they were trying to change. They fell into a past neural pathway, gaining comfort with foods that cause an inflammatory response, which led to pain, not sleeping, and not exercising, which led to more family and career frustrations.

Think of your thoughts as a cascade of events. Which way do you want the cascade to flow? You have control and a choice regarding every thought, so make it good. Let your Belief become knowing and your knowing become being.

Remember:
Whether you think you can or not, you're right.

No matter your thoughts, positive or negative, they are only thoughts. When we let these thoughts affect our behavior and actions, we begin to see other issues arise. I knew that I felt worse or had a relapse with my MS when stressed. In order to get a handle on the stress and recurring feeling that I was not enough, I had to reframe the thought into one that said I am and *know* that change was going to take time and practice.

Give yourself the patience and love to make these changes in your life. Change can be difficult, especially when you have practiced another way for a long time. You have an opportunity to practice a new way, and the new way can lead to you feeling better than you ever knew you could.

It was not easy at first, and the challenge came when I became hypersensitive to every muscle ache, shake, and occurrence of "feeling out of balance." When I would sweat too much at night or stumble when I stood up to walk. I had to begin adopting a new mantra and Believe I was okay, no matter what.

Yes, there were many times when I felt myself slip into an old negative thought pattern. These times became moments of Awareness and identified the triggers that caused my regression. I used these moments to identify the preceding events, activity, and even the foods that I ate. As I began to adjust the activity or eliminate the foods that I recognized as causing the response, I began to change. Over time, the positive thoughts and actions became automatic, and I began feeling better. The incidences of MS decreased, and I began controlling the stress that caused the relapse and poor feeling.

> Changing a mindset takes time,
> practice, patience, and self-love.
> Allow yourself the freedom of making this shift; it
> is a gift you give yourself.
> Take care of yourself during these changes.

Recognize critical thoughts quickly and replace them with fresh, positive ones. Over time, you will begin to notice your positive thoughts become automatic. Maybe someday, you will look in the mirror and not recognize the empowered person that stands in front of you.

Believe—Know—BE.

Chapter 9

Healing Behaviors

"Understand that the right to choose your own path is a sacred privilege. Use it. Dwell in possibility."

– Oprah Winfrey, *"What Oprah Knows for Sure About Freedom"*

Early on, the TIAs (Transient Ischemic Attacks), which were the brief stroke-like attacks, happened randomly.

I remember being in Breckenridge, Colorado, skiing with my dad and son. Yes, I was still skiing, and it was terrifying. I could not stop thinking about rocketing down the hill and having one of my episodes. Of course, this actually happened. I was fortunate enough that, after thirty years of skiing, I could stop when I began to notice it. I waited it out, which took about ten seconds, but it was still scary as hell.

One evening, as we walked home after going out for dinner, which was only a mile and a half from the house we were staying at, I was forced to stop multiple times. I learned humility, as I sat in front of my dad and son. They wondered if I was going to be okay each time.

These attacks were all I could think about, which brought more fear than the paralyzed leg and MS diagnosis (years later) combined. Every time I stood up or moved for long distances, I would feel the sensation that a TIA was starting. When one struck, an odd tingling sensation began creeping from my head, down my spine, and flooded the right side of my body, leaving me with little functioning and a feeling of being "locked in place." They stopped my ability to walk, think, and function normally for about ten seconds.

I hid these attacks from everyone and became good at anticipating each episode. I created strategies so those around me were not aware of them, and as far as I knew, no one who was not close to me knew about them. I became good at masking and deflecting a conversation, giving myself the needed few seconds to recover. My loved ones knew and so did my business partner.

During this time, I started to notice something: A correlation between stress and the frequency of the TIAs. The challenge was that I was under a lot of stress.

As my fear rose, I wondered, "Is this just a snapshot/demo of what my death will be like?"

Morbid, I know, but at that time, I felt the depth of what was happening, out of my control. I began believing in a possible new reality that was not good. Although my thoughts and beliefs were changed by each TIA, I knew there had to be a reason. I wanted control and used my past experiences of the paralyzed leg to give me hope that I would find a way. I began to look at every correlating factor that caused them, like stress, sleep, what I ate and drank, along with certain activities I performed. The awareness of what made me feel better or worse became an experiment in certain behaviors and actions. As I discovered what was working for me, my Belief of being able to overcome this fearful time in my life slowly grew, and new behaviors and habits emerged.

Doctors do not make this easier, and at times, neither does family, both of whom should be your advocates, cheerleaders, and support team. During my "episodes" if I heard someone say, "You know what you should do…" and give me another piece of advice, I was going to lose it. They did not have to feel the fear or the episodes, nor did they have the realization that I was not the same person I once thought I was.

Right after the episodes began, it was difficult to dislodge Who I Thought I Was, even though my mindset was working hard at doing so. I was anchored in my identity as an athlete, All-American Triathlete, Ironman, and the guy who lost eighty-five pounds to accomplish it all.

Due to this engrained mindset and identity, I was still at CrossFit five times per week, skiing, biking, and trying to run. I had just finished Ironman a few years before, and the identity of being an Ironman was stronger than any poor feeling or episode. I held on to it so tightly that I could feel it slip through my fingers. With each episode, I felt that my identity was getting on a train and leaving. I did not know if it would come back, and I so desperately wanted the "old me" back.

In my pursuit to maintain my current identity, I studied and knew I needed to heal the TIAs as soon as possible. It was now one hundred percent up to me, and I liked it, because I felt like I was in control, again. I used this budding identity and mindset that I was smart enough to research and experiment as the new seed in my mind. I was open-minded, following threads and rabbit trails as I continued to understand why the TIAs were happening. I became engrossed, slowly, into new ideas and behaviors, like meditation along with a consistent pre and probiotic regimen, which worked to replace my gut microbiome.

Over the next few months, I saw improvements. I viewed my body like a science experiment. I knew what I was doing was not harmful: I was using food to create improvement. My desire not to live with the TIAs and knowing what I wanted blended with Who I Was. This evolved into the drive needed to have a mindset of possibility.

What was my alternative?

These moments and shifts came slowly, and I followed the trails of success. These trails were easy to recognize, because each one lessened the amount of TIAs and made me feel better. After three months, the TIAs stopped. I stopped taking the statin drug. If I had given up, been a victim, and thought I was not smarter than doctors, then I would still be taking the statin and experiencing the TIAs. Who knows what would have happened if I continued living with the fear of the episodes?

When we feel like we are losing control, our desire may be to gain that control back and stop living in the unknown. The only way that you'll actually feel more empowered and like you have control is if you begin to act and behave in ways that cause you to heal, rather than acting and behaving in ways that continue to focus on your suffering. This means making conscious choices to confront your triggers of fear and stress, and it also means making conscious choices about how to improve your mood and habits.

> We must dive into the fact that all day-to-day behaviors lead to choices that can be healing, if they're promoting a healthy life.

Beginning of the Day

What is the first thing you tell yourself when you wake up in the morning? Do you have a mantra or statement you declare to yourself that brings a sense of possibility?

Often, we wake up in the morning with little intention of choosing how we want to wake up and what we intend for the day ahead. For example, my intention is to begin each day with meditation, journaling my thoughts, journaling what I am grateful for, and then read and write my personal affirmations.

Although I try to start my day with these beautiful practices, life happens— an unexpected phone call, oversleeping, or some other unanticipated event keeps me away from my practice, some days. In these moments, I have a choice of letting my good intention spin me in a downward spiral of guilt, or I can choose to give myself grace and love myself in these moments, reminding myself that I am human and things happen. Self-love in these moments will keep stress where it should be; self-love in these moments allows for awareness and the lessons it teaches.

These first thoughts and feelings set the tone for the day. Often, we tell ourselves the day is going to be busy, long, and difficult, then we follow those thoughts with thoughts of, "I can't..." or "I am not..." You fill in the rest of the statements with your own negative dialogue.

We have choices about how we want to be and which behaviors and actions we perform. In most cases, no one tells you how you are supposed to think and be when you wake up.

When I was out of shape, eating pizza and drinking beer when I was younger, I started my day out with negative thoughts, thinking that I was not enough, which led to a feeling and actions of defeat. I tried to numb these feelings by overeating and drinking, which led to the results of being stressed out and overweight. When I decided to change my life, I started by changing my morning routine and what I told myself when I woke up.

The morning routine started with experiments with food, sleep, and mitigating stress. I paid attention to what my day was like and gave each experiment at least two weeks. I looked at how I felt, what happened around me and what I was attracting, and what my behaviors were. Was I sad? Happy? Fearful?

Most of the time, it was not easy. It felt like I picked up a new job, and that was when knowing What I Wanted in my life served me. The trial-and-error process meant that the decision-fatigue struggle was real, but I had to go through it, guided by a beacon of light that kept me moving forward.

When I had a good day, I altered my morning routine to follow the mindset, behaviors, and actions that created that day.

When we start anything new, we start with small steps. For example, when I was two-hundred fifty-five pounds, out of shape, and a sedentary guy, my thoughts were about getting through the day, going to work, chores that needed to be done, etc. I never thought about working out or trying to change anything. When I had a thought about not being that way, I had feelings of shame. I had negative thoughts when looking in the mirror. So, I used that as a starting point of change.

I had allowed the feeling of "being fat," and thoughts of "I need to lose weight" to fester. I reframed these thoughts from shameful ones to ones reminding me about the next step. When the new, larger pants I bought felt tight, I reminded myself of my goals, allowing the moment to act as motivation about what I did *not* want.

At the beginning, it was far-fetched to think and believe that running, exercise, or waking up early to do any of those activities were "fun" or even possible. If you would have asked me right out of college if I was a runner, I would have laughed as I took another bite of pizza. I did not have a reason to start running, biking, or doing any other activity. It was not until I had a reason that a new thought began. I needed a reason to think differently about myself, every day. Only then did I slowly change. The reasons that became possibilities and drove me forward included living a longer life for my growing family and a desire to not be the way I was. When I woke in the morning, my thoughts slowly began to shift to: "I am in shape and healthy."

What could I do easily to take the first step toward reaching what I wanted? At the time, instead of jumping into exercise and running, I began with my thoughts. That small step led to another, and then another. During the journey of my athletic accomplishments, no one could see how they developed but me. This journey began a little at a time, then all of a sudden. I started to feel and see my life changing to what I wanted, and it brought hope. This hope led to a gradual shift of doing just 1 percent more each day.

When we try to take too large of a leap toward What We Want, it can become easy to get discouraged. It can take one moment of discouragement to derail the new intention and path you are on. If I set a goal to run one more minute the next day, it is not hard to wrap my mind around sixty seconds. As the change slowly begins to happen, we feel and hear the encouragement we give ourselves, and our behaviors begin to shift to possibility. For example, I had the identity of being an All-American Triathlete and marathon runner, then my mindset (what I think when I wake up) reinforced the belief that I was an athlete. Then, running and biking were not hard; I didn't perceive them as "things I cannot do." The mindset of *enjoying* running and biking drives the behavior and the desire that makes me want to run and bike more.

You do not have to be an athlete. The best place to start is where you are right now on your journey. Take small steps toward What You Want, and celebrate the wins regularly, no matter what they are. Pay attention to your behavior, because those behaviors can be the guideposts for lessons that you are meant to learn. Do not forget about your own love and compassion, for that is the grace that you desperately need sometimes.

Starting the change becomes the challenge. Our old habits, thoughts, and actions are known. It is much easier to continue an old habit or thought, even if it is not serving you. Stepping into an unknown future can lead to anxiety and stress, and our Ego may begin telling us all the reasons we can't. We use our past to justify our choice of not changing.

I am too fat. I have had two knee surgeries. I am too busy. This has never worked anyhow...

These can all be excuses that your Ego may use to keep you from the perceived unfounded dangers of the unknown. Use these thoughts as reasons for making change. Go back to Who You Are and your reason for What You Want and make *those* your motivation. Start with small shifts, like writing one positive affirmation that has meaning for you on a Post-it note and putting it on your bathroom mirror. Be aware of how you feel in each moment, not dwelling on whether the thought or feeling is good or bad; just become aware of those thoughts and feelings.

Chapter 9 Exercise

Recognizing Patterns of Behavior

Behavior is what we do and what we don't do. It is the direct outcome of knowing Who You Are and your mindset. Both of these must transform to drive and achieve the behavior to heal. Our behavior is 100 percent in our control. We are what we repeatedly do and don't do. Our behavior is critical because it impacts the actions we take.

In your journal ask yourself these questions and write down your answers:

- What is my current Behavior? or What are my current patterns of Behavior?
    - Example: *I am worried, which has me eating fast food.* (the behavior)
- What Behavior must I model for myself in order to heal?
    - Example: *Joy and love, making the choice to eat fruits and vegetables*
- What is the one positive behavior I am going to start right now?
- What is one negative behavior I am going to stop right now?

This is a journey that starts slowly. Be okay when old patterns of behavior show up, just be aware of them. How long have your current behavior patterns been present in your life? You will find it has been a long time that you have practiced them; they are ingrained in your habits and thoughts. Give yourself the grace to begin making a change.

Overcoming Excuses

It is important to begin taking action now. I am the master at excuses and justifying every one of them. It is easy to *not* work out, *not* meditate because we are too busy, or eat the same unhealthy processed foods even though you know they make you feel worse. We are creatures of habit, and we do not want to change, even though the only constant in the world is change. You began to change the minute you were born and have continued to do so. Change does not have to be a radical shift even though it can be. Over time, small almost unnoticeable changes can create a new you. So, to begin moving the other way, start with one slight shift of attention. Use the new way of Who You Want to Be to begin shifting your habits. Relish the celebration of small wins.

During this journey, I have had the pleasure of meeting and coaching some incredible people toward their new realities of not being *defined* by their disease but *thriving*, instead. I remember an incredible gentleman in nursing school who came to me due to family struggles and frustrations occurring because of his MS diagnosis. During our first conversation, he proclaimed to me that he did not meditate or take the time to slow down. The most he had done at this point was adjust his diet, exercise, and attend his church services.

Deep down, he knew there had to be a way to shift his negative behavior and thoughts. He knew what he wanted but needed help seeing the first step. We uncovered what he valued and the triggers that caused stress that could derail his progress. We used his desire to be a great dad, and an even better husband, to fuel the change that he wanted.

During the journey, I was witness to his discovery of the beautiful Self that he was, as he became more comfortable slowing down and going within during meditation. During the first steps, it would have been easy to stop and go back to the old habits of thought that led to the life he did not want. After a little bit of time, he began being the dad and person he desired to be, filled with love and joy of the little moments that life gives us.

As his joy grew slowly, he began feeling better, and he began understanding and controlling his symptoms. During one of our calls, he told me a story of how he taught a woman before surgery to meditate and calm herself. She was experiencing a massive amount of stress and anxiety prior to the surgery. After teaching her to breathe and meditate through the experience, she began to feel better. The surgery went well. As he told me the story, I had tears in my eyes as I thought of the difference he was making for others, simply because he decided to change his reality and behavior. Today, this gentleman has seen his body heal; after undergoing another MRI, his report shows decreased brain and spinal lesions. His doctors have proclaimed that the MS is burned out.

Hearing stories of others who shifted their own realities into possibilities motivates me to lean into the power of this work. When our own possibilities are realized, there is not much that can stop us from creating the lives we want, no matter what happened to us.

Chapter 9 Exercise

Replacing Negative Thoughts

The next time your mind wanders, leading toward negative thoughts and fears, become aware of the thought and replace the thought with love. Imagine a time when you felt love. This could have been from your spouse, friend, or even your best canine friend. Do you see yourself as healed? What are you doing, saying, and being when you are healed?

In your journal, write down what your life is like now that you overcame your disease.

- How do you feel?
- What are your emotions?
- What are you doing?
- Where are you living?
- What does your house look like?
- What are your current habits?
- Who is in your life?
- What are you cooking? Can you smell and taste it?
- How much love do you feel for yourself?

Put yourself in the space as if it already happened. Because it *has* already happened!

Take your time with this exercise and imagine yourself as healed. Live *now* as if it is so, no matter how you feel today. Practice this habit *twice per day*, once in the morning when you wake, and another time in the evening, before you go to bed.

Chapter 9 Exercise
Measure & Track New Healing Behavior

Begin measuring and tracking the results from your new healing behavior. For me, I used to be able to walk only 900 steps (yes, I counted them) when I was experiencing equilibrium and walking motor-control issues. My goal every two weeks was to walk one hundred more steps until I could walk a mile.

These small wins not only kept my little voice at bay but also fueled hope and more positive thought. These small wins led me to keep trying and exploring how good I could feel.

> Try something new that
> leads toward What You Want.
> For example, something like learning
> to cook, garden, or shop for healthy food.

Chapter 9 Exercise
Develop Your Curiosity

Take action on one thing to heal. What is the one thing you are going to begin telling yourself? For example, I am smart enough to begin reading and studying food as medicine. This thought could lead to a behavior of curiosity. You may find yourself at the bookstore in the alternative healing section. You may decide to buy the book and begin reading it. This book may lead to another, and then another. You may begin buying different foods at the grocery store, and the cycle continues.

If this seems daunting, remember
Who You Are and What You Want. Let these be
the gasoline or push you need to take action.
You can always go for a walk and think about it.
Just start with one small step or thought
right now, because *you* are worth it.

Chapter 10

Healed/New Identity

> "The ego is only an illusion, but a very influential one. Letting the ego-illusion become your identity can prevent you from knowing your true self. Ego, the false idea of believing that you are what you have or what you do, is a backwards way of assessing and living life."
>
> – Wayne Dyer, *"The Ego Illusion"*

I stood in the shower, surveying the event. I had picked up a heavy load of snow. I felt intense pain in my lower spine, and I could not support myself on the toes of my right foot. Before I could finish surveying the entirety of what happened, the fear set in. The fear of my life changing drastically washed over me. Would I ever run again? Would I ever compete again?

I could feel fear drain my hope, and the loud negative voice started: "You are broken. You will never race again. Why did you do that?"

It went on and on. With my next breath, I buried the fear deep within me. I did not want to face the reality. It was easier to run away from this fear than to address it, and I ran away from it. If it had not been for some kind individuals (angels) in my life, I may be still running from it today.

I felt like my thoughts were a bowl of spaghetti, not connecting, and scattered. As I began to review my options, resources, and what I thought were possible solutions, I felt like I needed to take control, so I gripped my life tighter. I tried to use my past experiences of working harder and putting my head down to "grind it out" to push through and make my leg work again. As I gripped tighter to my old self, the reality and hope of making my leg work again drifted farther away, which led to the cascading spiral downward, toward a deep depression.

After viewing the experience with hindsight, I have realized that "the way out is through." Even with the storm life presented to me. Going through the storm did not mean pushing harder; it meant sitting still and surrendering to something bigger than myself.

Priorities

My identity was key in knowing how decisions would be made, as more and more of them were presented. I made the things that were important to me a priority and made some difficult decisions. I elevated my curiosity and allowed myself time and made room for the desire to research. As I was continually approaching these scary and unknown moments, avoidance and denial crept in. My thought process at the time was that if I ignored the situation, then it could not be happening to me.

I started the slow journey between feeling like a victim and being in denial, which led to listening and following those who I felt had superior knowledge but not necessarily our highest and best desires. This way of thinking can lead to fewer choices and a myopic viewpoint that this suggestion is the only way. We start to limit our choices without knowing what all the choices are. We may begin to justify the reason why we did not research, change behaviors, or understand the dangers and options further.

Remember whatever is decided by you is right, but you may find that you beat yourself up over any choice you have made. Understanding and working through the should haves and negative thoughts, learning from the choices you made so you can make a different one can be key during this time. Understanding and accepting Who We Are and What We Want can help us craft our new identity. The choices we make can either lead us to our new healthy identity or enable the avoidance and continue hiding from ourselves and the fear.

You are on a journey, and just like a road trip, you follow a map, or at least, you follow the general directions of North, South, East, or West. You pick a direction, and you start moving. If I want to visit California, I am not going to get there by sitting at home dreaming of California. I have to take action on the first step, and that will lead me to another choice—one that may have more options or choices. This first step may also lead you to feeling better, understanding the beautiful soul you are.

Putting New Visualizations into Practice

After paralyzing my leg, I knew what I wanted and did not want when it came to fixing my leg, which was no longer working. Orthopedic doctors were a last resort, due to the stories I heard of surgeries gone wrong—surgeries where rods are inserted and screws are placed in the spine, screwing two opposing discs together, called a "spinal fusion." At the time, I knew a few people suffering from back pain due to a spinal fusion, and the surgery did not look like it went as expected.

My past identity as an athlete was still primary, and I was not about to give that up, so I gripped tighter. Running and competing in triathlons again became my next challenge. I had not sustained an injury that required surgery for more than fifteen years, and it was not going to happen again. As my desire for what I wanted became stronger and blended with the identity of being a competitive athlete, I was open to trying and listening to what was around me.

As the months went by, I noticed my mindset shift to the negative. A feeling and belief that I could possibly never do what I loved began to creep in. It was slow at first, then as time passed, so did the thought that this could be permanent. As the thought of the severity of my accident crept over me, the choices I made to try to fix my leg seemed logical at the time. I could not see past step one, and I was petrified of continuing down this path because I didn't know where it led.

Was I going to become the guy that always had back problems? Was I going to live perpetually in the past, while "Glory Days" by Bruce Springsteen played in my head as my new theme song? All I could think about was loss and scarcity. At the time, I had no control over the little voice in my head.

Prior to the paralyzed leg, I was building my race plan and was living in the possibility of how I was going to finish an ultramarathon and then Ironman, as well as making it a pursuit to beat my fastest half-Ironman time, on my way to achieving All-American Triathlete status again. I had nothing limiting me before the injury, but life became dramatically different with one shovelful of heavy snow and with every painful step I took. All my plans changed, and my new plans were filled with scarcity, as I realized that running was impossible.

This feeling of scarcity was one that I had not felt in a long time. No matter the diagnosis or injury, our minds can easily slip into what we do not have, reinforced by our current reality. These feelings of lack and scarcity can only attract more lack and scarcity. If we tell ourselves that we "cannot," then our thoughts become our reality because we are not willing to listen to any depth of possibility. Our mindset, energy, and behaviors required do not start leading us down the road of small steps to recovery and thoughts of being healed. During this time our positive thoughts are critical, and sometimes, this is all we have.

Healing Actions Make a Healed Identity

At this time, I had worked for over thirty years crafting my identity. I was proud of being an athlete, I had lost eighty-five pounds, and in four years, I made a designation of All-American triathlete. I was proud of who I was and felt like my life was on the right path. But once it was all taken away, I could not see past the next move, as fear began to dictate how I operated. For me, I was no longer a fiercely competitive triathlete. I was a guy with a back injury who could not walk without a limp.

So, I started with chiropractors and tried everything I could, from Active Release Therapy, to spinal decompression, and many more approaches. As I became open to looking at other angles to heal my leg, more options presented themselves because I was open to hearing them.

As I met with my doctors, I could have been told anything; all the advice and wisdom sounded like white noise. As I look back years later, I can see where my blind spots were and what I chose to ignore. I chose to ignore the fact that my leg was not improving, and also ignore the subtle suggestions my doctors gave me to look at different approaches, like alternative surgeries that did not include spinal fusion.

I did not want to face my new reality. This new reality was foreign, and because of it, the new negative mindset quickly followed. If you asked me at the time, I could not answer two simple questions: Who I Was and What I Wanted. If you told me everything happens for a reason, you may have been punched, or at the least, given a dirty look. I began to flail and grab at anything. I did not like this new feeling of not being good enough or this new negative mindset that engulfed me. Instead of focusing on what I wanted, I focused on what I could *not* do, which led to depression.

What are you holding on to?

No matter what you are holding on to, it is valid and very real. This self-perception drives our well-being and choices. Even though we may feel that we have little or no choice, the act of not making a choice is still a choice. When your sense of self or your identity is suddenly taken away, you can be left with fear, loss, change, and the anxiety of the unknown. We do not always look at this forced slowdown as positive, but we always have a choice about our own self-perception, and no one can take that away.

The first step is addressing this negative mindset, and I was forced to look at my reactions and choices differently. I could have very easily gone numb in front of the doctors and taken their advice as the "only way." Instead, I remained open to choices and did not let fear dictate my next step.

Any choice you have made is the right choice, because you made it, and making a choice (no matter how small) can be better than making no choice at all. We overcome our fears through action, and to be shown other potential options, we may need to move slightly to see our situation from a different angle. At your current predicament or situation, you may feel there is not a good choice. During this time, remember—by sitting quietly and listening to your higher Self, by quieting the busy judgmental mind, you can make the best choice possible.

So, what happens when we blindly make choices and any amount of fear is blended with it? We do not like to admit that the choice was made blindly out of fear, so we justify our reasons. Some of our choices, based on our situation, can lead us to depression, stress, and anger.

A New Focus

It is important during this time to turn in and focus on yourself. We can be so caught up in our situation and the rapid or fearful choices we have to make that we forget Who We Are. The negative Ego and fearful mind can keep us from seeing the most important parts of the experience. This important part is easy to ignore and hide from, due to the external situation being so loud that we cannot hear. This critical, most important part is *you*.

As we take time to quiet our egos and fears, we hear another voice that is filled with compassion and love. As we forgive and offer compassion to ourselves for what may have happened, we take responsibility for our situation. This responsibility, under the direction of our own compassion and love, leads us to forgiveness. As our forgiveness grows within ourselves, gratitude for Who We Are and where we are emerges. These moments can be difficult to see right now, but the only way out is through the storm you are in. At the end of the storm is peace, where you can surrender and know that you are living your highest and best, as the lessons and Awareness of Self come into focus.

Chapter 10 Exercise

"I Am" Statements

The work you did earlier in the book is going to serve you now. Take the work you have done regarding Who You Are and What You Want. What words are commonly appearing as you look at both? Are you kind and want to help others? Are you active? Are you a loving grandfather/grandmother who wants to play with your grandkids? By looking at these correlations, group them together into new statements about yourself that start with I am:

- I am a survivor.
- I am smart.
- I am loving.
- I am possible.
- I am joy.

What would you tell your spouse, friend, family, and a doctor about Who You Are? What do you tell yourself?

As you make your list of "I am" statements, focus on the internal aspects and Values that make up Who You Are, (for example: *love, joy, driven*, etc.) instead of the external factors that can change, like *athlete, wealthy, teacher, mother, grandparent*, etc.

By the time I went into the doctor, I had already decided my game plan of curiosity, and I understood all that I could about my situation. I knew that worrying and doing only what the doctor suggested did not serve my identity, and it was not Who I Was or What I Wanted. My choice to be curious and understand everything I could was non-negotiable.

This was my life, and I wanted my grandkids to know the love and joy of their grandpa, even though at that time, I was many years away from that experience.

Conclusion

Our lives are filled with many choices, with some being easy while others seem impossible. During these choices, we have the option to make ourselves into anyone we want. We try to make these choices with open eyes, wisdom, and education.

During this time, focus on you and what your higher Self may be leading you to. This does not mean ignoring all the experts and advice given to you. I am not suggesting you put others on a pedestal above your own wisdom and knowledge. This external validation of our choices can keep us from looking inward for our answers, ignoring sometimes the most important part, which is ourselves.

Our higher Self always has our highest and best as its priority, but we have to be open to listening to it. Slowing down and trusting ourselves can be the most important work you do. Slowing down does not mean stopping or freezing your actions; it means slowing down enough to be aware of your surroundings and feelings. How you feel during this time—internally, at the gut level—can be some of the greatest wisdom you receive.

> Listen to your intuition and higher Self. Ask to be open enough to hear what is not being said. You are amazing. Do not let others dim your brilliant light. Let your light shine forth so you can heal and be the person you were meant to be.

Chapter 11

Small Steps/The Essential Nature of all Progress

> Be not afraid of growing slowly, be afraid only of standing still.
>
> – Chinese Proverb, *Common Chinese Proverbs Revealed and Explained*

Priorities

Many times in my life, I have felt stuck. Instead of taking a small step in any direction, I stood frozen and justified my reason. *The time was not right. I was tired. I did not like my options.* I could write a book on excuses, but they are just that: excuses. Out of my own fear of failure and feeling like I was not enough, I felt frozen in place, as fear washed over me. My mood and fear clouded my judgment, and at times, I found myself avoiding the change or taking any action to change my feeling and situation. I decided to focus on the big moves that could get me where I wanted to go, instead of the small moves that got me unstuck.

For example, imagine you could not eat for forty-eight hours. Your hunger may affect your mood, and your primary desire may be to eat something, anything. When you are given the opportunity to eat, you find the time to eat—no matter how busy, tired, or distracted you are. The steps you take and the speed at which you take action depend on your reasons for eating, no matter how hungry you were and how strong the desire was.

Did you want to eat alone or with family? Did you have the energy or time to make food, or did you think having an organic carrot with hummus would suffice? Were you thinking about satisfying the urge to eat right now, or were you thinking about the future and the desire to plant an apple tree so this hunger would not happen again?

Your general feeling drove the actions necessary to no longer be hungry in the short term, and possibly, the future.

If I wanted something I did not have in my life, I had a choice to take a step forward or not. If I decided to take a step, I would move through these small steps, aware of my emotional well-being as my barometer of purpose. If, at any time, I became stuck or crossed an area where no action was taken due to avoidance or excuses, I looked at where I was stuck and made the step smaller. I tried to learn from the lack of action forward and understand why, with no judgment or ridicule. If I did not move forward, what was I not listening to, or was I not aware of the gap in importance and desire?

Like the example above, the desire to eat and knowing how gave you options so you could take steps to satisfy this desire. Anything with a high level of importance is made a priority, and it gets done. But what happens when we do not see any type of step forward? When we feel lost, and we may not be able to see the small step that is right in front of us. The obvious can become clouded, leaving us thinking about the big outcome desired. The sometimes-obsessive thoughts of the bigger desire can leave us feeling ungrateful for the small things that lead us to the desired outcome.

Breaking Your Big Plan into Smaller Steps

When I woke up the morning following signing up for Ironman, I first reacted with the thought, "What have I done?"

My decision was intentional, and I knew what I was getting into. The emotion and reason for signing up directly stemmed from being fed up with the progress of healing my paralyzed leg, and I justified my decision logically.

What were the facts? I had not raced in a multi-sport event for three years. I engaged in physical therapy and ran a little. I did spend the summer on my bike, attempting rides like the ascent of Mt. Evans—a 14,264-foot peak that can be accessed with a paved road, but it involved more than sixty miles of riding and a 8,464-feet cycling ascent from my house.

I had maintained a little endurance but nowhere near where I needed to be to finish Ironman. I knew what I needed to do to improve my leg, in order to finish Ironman, and I had 364 days to do it. I knew that blindly going out and conducting long rides, runs, and swims was not going to get me across the finish line. In the past, I used to call unplanned miles, "junk miles." I needed a plan, and then, I needed to follow it. I had books galore, and the internet was a wealth of knowledge, along with my experience from the past. I also had good friends who had competitively raced in Ironmans that I could call on.

This small first step—recognizing that I needed a plan before I laced up any shoe—was not easy. The act of the event was easy once you had trained, but the mental strength to *not* react was the hard part. When we have made a choice, no matter what is decided, we inherently want to take action on our decision immediately. This immediate action, although laden with good intention, falls down after the newness wears off. Our adrenaline from signing up to a big endeavor, or the hope that what we are doing will get us past a proverbial finish line, can be dismantled with our negative ego mind.

Your success for anything comes with steps, whether you have been aware of them or not. As human beings, we tend to think linearly—one step after another, in a straight, direct fashion. For example, imagine your education, as you went from kindergarten through high school, each year building onto the one before. When we finish school, we are told to find work, eventually find love, have kids, raise a family, and then retire. As we go through life, these linear events do not always follow a straight trajectory. It is more common that the events and trajectory of our lives is like a winding path, with many twists and turns. During our journey, if we are diagnosed with a disease or experience a tragic event, the straight path can turn abruptly, leaving us feeling lost and stuck. This does not mean a plan is not needed, but the key is to remain flexible in the plan you made.

I love the dialogue between Alice and the Cheshire cat from the book, *Alice in Wonderland,* by Lewis Carroll:

"Would you tell me, please, which way I ought to go from here?" asked Alice.

"That depends a good deal on where you want to get to," said the Cat.

"I don't much care where—" said Alice.

"Then it doesn't matter which way you go," said the Cat.

When we do not have a plan, it can feel like we are tossed about with every bad feeling, idea, or piece of information and advice. During this time, it is important to know where you are going and what your finish line is. As you think about and research possible steps to get there, break them down into smaller steps that encourage you to keep moving forward; it is critical to create movement. If I had started Ironman training with a sixty-mile bike ride and followed it with a ten-mile run, I most likely would not have made it to the next day of training.

In my past, I remember moments when I was full of ambition and drive, only to have the excuses creep in. The "I'll just" mentality was crippling: *I'll just do two workouts tomorrow. I'll just ride a little farther*, etc.

I had the same ideas and reasons, and I knew what I wanted. My reason and desire were not enough. I had to create internal, ongoing motivation to keep taking the small steps forward. To keep the negative mind at bay, our plan should be laced with small success, and sometimes, the act of waking up to train was enough for the small success needed.

For example, I had a reason beyond myself when I created the goal for this book—I wanted to inspire others to take the first step toward Belief, in order to heal whatever ails them. I told people about it, notified people on social media, in hopes that social accountability would create consistent action. I hoped this was all the motivation needed to complete the book you now read, but it was not. I had written a discombobulated, unorganized stream of consciousness. Yes, it was a good start that fizzled quickly. After five years of staring at the words I had written, my Self-Awareness and deep work on myself understanding my purpose and Who I Was led to self-encouragement and knowing that I was *enough* to be an author.

> Sometimes, when we feel stuck,
> the smaller we make the steps, the easier it can
> be to move forward. Sitting with yourself quietly
> and going deeper into the work of discovering you
> can be the most important first step. As we step
> into the Awareness of ourselves, be open to
> listening and be aware of inspiration,
> as you are *creating* the small steps forward.

As we take these steps with no judgment, we offer ourselves the patience and grace needed to take small steps. Ensure that part of your plan includes the Awareness of knowing Who You Are, as discussed in previous chapters, so you can access them when times get difficult.

The Curse of "I'll Just"

The curse of "I'll Just" was always there. Have you ever meant to do something new and said the words "I'll just," either out loud or to yourself?

I'll just wake up earlier tomorrow. I'll just write longer tomorrow. I'll just eat a healthier dinner tomorrow.

I had to make the decision whether I was going to write a book or not. When I decided this is what I wanted to accomplish, then I could take steps to complete it. Like the steps taken and learned from walking the path to control MS, I knew I had to take a small, easily achievable step to keep the curse of "I'll just" at bay.

The achievable first step was key to creating momentum. So, I did the logical thing anyone would do when they have no idea what to do or how to get started: I Googled it.

"How to write a book" is what I searched—rudimentary and basic, I know, but it was a step. I was not about to let the little voice tell me how I was not qualified or how stupid my first step was. It is easy, during this fragile time, to "self-reject" and kill your own momentum before it gets started. I knew I would search the phrase and that would lead me to another step. These steps were not difficult, and they took minutes to complete. Some of these steps were taken as I waited to pick up my kids from school. I allowed curiosity to continue the flow of my forward direction. These first steps led me to building a writing plan with small daily deliverables that I began to enjoy.

I had no idea how I was going to do it, but I did not need to. As we discussed before, "You do not have to see the whole staircase, just the first step."

I did not realize the importance of one small, seemingly insignificant step. Our steps, no matter how small, should encourage us and have a completion date assigned to them, to keep the thought of "I'll just" under control. After succeeding at the first step, begin thinking about and looking for the next step. The next steps can seem elusive and distant when I think about the end. Our desire pushes us further away from the possibility of achievement and self-encouragement to keep moving.

As you move down the path—one small step after another—pay attention to how you feel inside. As human beings, we have the beautiful ability to *feel*. Our bodies and our general feelings can be the guidepost needed for knowing and taking action on the next step.

When was the last time you had to make a decision and had a bad feeling about it? This feeling, and awareness of it, can lead us to thinking about a new direction or researching other options. If we disregard this feeling, we may be ignoring another possible option. As you are eating the proverbial elephant one bite at a time, be aware of whether the thought is from the negative Ego, warning us of danger that is unfounded. This thought could lead you to understanding the negative voice that has kept you from your desire.

Often, we think of the next step as physical action, instead of slowing down and going in. Many times, when writing this book, my ego kept telling me that what I was writing was not enough; someone more qualified than I should write this book. If I would have listened to this inner voice, I would have stopped writing.

Sometimes, the next step can be one within as we work our plan. Paying attention to how I felt on a daily basis became a small step of self-encouragement. Was I happy or upset? How many times did the little voice try to step in? What was I not listening to?

> This step, no matter how small and insignificant, was first taken with the intention to complete it.

No Task Is Impossible

The weight and grandiosity given to seemingly impossible tasks, or to a diagnosis, freezes action and leaves you in a holding pattern, looking for the perfect runway to land on. As we are on our own paths, we realize that it is not about finding the perfect runway; it's about the importance of landing the plane before it runs out of gas.

Instead of thinking about how large and impossible the task is, focus on how to simplify it and what is needed to take the first step. For example, if you want to cook something extravagant for your family during the holidays, you don't approach the task by looking at the raw ingredients, then just trying to "go for it." If you are a trained chef, you might, but your training has already given you the confidence and skills. If you are feeling overwhelmed, you might first look up a recipe or try to remember a meal or experience you had. As you are giving yourself the thought of possibility that you can do this, you may practice before the event.

You begin cooking, looking at the next step—which may be to sauté an onion. When you look at the raw onion, you may need to peel it and chop it before sautéing it. This large task, broken down into small, successful steps, keeps you moving. The success of completing the small steps keeps you moving toward the end goal of what you want, which is a gourmet homemade meal. These small tasks distract our minds from being overwhelmed by the large, desired outcome we want to achieve. Sometimes, the distractions and excuses of the large task justify our reasons for not moving forward. This moment is a defining moment, when we are faced with the fear and unknown of a disease. We are given a choice to move forward or not, and both are okay, if they align to Who You Are and What You Want.

When I was first diagnosed, I was afraid of the potential disability MS might leave my body in. I wanted to heal MS and live symptom free, but the problem was, I had no idea where to start. Instead of thinking about all the reasons why it would be impossible, I broke down the steps into what I needed for the next step. Like Ironman and its training, I knew it was not one bike ride that got you across the finish line but a series of seemingly insignificant intentional steps, consistently completed over and over, that got you across the finish line in under seventeen hours.

I approached overcoming the symptoms and reversing MS in a similar fashion. I began thinking about what is a seemingly unimportant step that I could complete right now. I thought about what was put in my path over the last thirty days and wrote down anything that stood out from my normal day to day: Conversations I had, books that stood out, and people I met. I then took this list and asked myself, "Would I be interested in knowing more about something on this list?"

> There was a phrase a mentor of mine used:
> When the student is ready, the teacher will appear.

For me, the teacher came in the form of books, which led to videos, meeting people, conferences, and to others who had healed MS and provided support. At times, I was asked how I progressed, and the answer had so many unique steps and situations. I enjoyed the question, even as it became difficult to answer.

I tried to identify what the first step was for me, and although I know my situation was unique, I have learned that the first step is unique for everyone. It will be unique for you, too.

Use the beginning chapters of this book as a possible step. When you find anything—no matter how small—ask yourself, "Am I curious enough to stop everything I am doing now to explore this small step?"

This small step will either lead to more curiosity or to a dead end. If it is a dead end, pick the next small step and try again. Even if your first attempt was a dead end, you learned something. Be curious about *why* you feel it is a dead end. Every minute of every day is there to teach you something. Whether we take the time to listen and pay attention to what we are being taught is up to us.

Chapter 11 Exercise

Getting Past Hurdles with Smaller Steps

Take the exercises conducted in earlier chapters and begin spending time with your answers. Some of your answers may resonate and leave you feeling hopeful, while others may leave you feeling overwhelmed. To overcome the hurdle of action, *now is the time of doing more by doing less.*

As you review your awareness and writing, underline the sections and words that leave you hopeful. Remove the desire to correct or adjust your answers if you're feeling overwhelmed. Sit quietly with yourself, thinking and breathing.

Ask yourself these questions

- What part of this phrase or word brings me hope?
- Where do I feel this within my body?
- What are the quiet, almost unnoticeable, thoughts that came up while thinking about what I wrote?

Write down these answers as a stream of consciousness, with no judgment or structure.

Did you become curious about what you wrote? Are you curious and excited about knowing a deeper understanding regarding a direction or general topic? Use these moments of curiosity as your next step.

Conclusion

Sometimes, our growth and the desire for What We Want comes to us in surprising ways. We are brought up thinking that the way to answer questions is by using logic and current beliefs. Although these can be very important, they are not the only way. We allow our logic and fear of the unknown to keep us from taking necessary action. We ignore the internal voice trying to make its presence known. We ignore inspiration and discredit it with the fear we live with. Our fear can leave us frozen and stuck.

The way out of this fear is *through* the fear, as we take our small steps to self-discovery. These small, sometimes insignificant choices and moments can be the key you were looking for. It is the surprise, joy, and feeling better—like we used to—that guides us on our path. Our experiences and choices, not the big leaps we take, determine the outcome of our lives. The surprise of seeing the "new you" who has changed, and discovery of this *beautiful*, new you, become the inspiration for others to follow.

Stopping and deciding not to move forward in any direction can become the curse of this moment. Decide today that you are not going to stop because you love yourself fully. Realize that you are worth every step.

Chapter 12

The Importance of Belief

"We judge [w]hat we see, with certain eyes . . . whereas we ought therefore to believe, *because* we cannot see . . . But you, beloved, who possess this faith, or who have begun now newly to have it, let it be nourished and increase in you. For as things temporal have come, so long before foretold, so will things eternal also come, which are promised."

~ Saint Augustine, Concerning Faith of Things Not Seen

Three weeks before I was diagnosed with MS, and after I was fired, I received a book in the mail. The book was *Medical Medium* by Anthony William. At the time, I had no idea why I received it. I had gone through some medical challenges—healing the paralyzed leg and the TIAs—but why did I receive the book now? I thought I was past all the medical struggles. I chalked it up to a book for my then-wife and never looked at it, because I had no need. At the time, I did not understand and was not aware of the future or what this book would mean to me. With hindsight, I can say that it was the first step, even though I had no idea there was a step to take.

Before my official diagnosis of MS, I went to my family doctor for a checkup and inquired about the dizzy, almost vertigo-like events I was experiencing. I walked out of the doctor's office, and I was not thinking about something worse or speculating about any type of disease. I thought it was stress related, and my body was trying to tell me something. After years of being a competitive athlete and sustaining prior injuries, I was attuned with my body. What came next was a surprise, or better said, a wake-up call with a 2x4 (or ten).

After my first MRI, I was notified by a nurse over the phone that I showed signs of multiple sclerosis. I had no idea what it was, so I Googled it and researched WebMD to begin educating myself on MS. As I read the stories about MS, the prognosis was not positive. What was a diagnosis like MS going to do to me?

I turned to *Medical Medium*, remembering there was a chapter on multiple sclerosis. I was looking for hope instead of the narrow viewpoint the doctors gave me, stating the worst case instead of hopeful options. I knew thinking about the limiting possibilities was only going to worry me and build negative thoughts. What did I know? Besides experiencing a few correlations like stress and what I ate. It seemed rudimentary, but that was all I had. At that point, I had lost my job and was diagnosed with MS in the same month. What was the Universe, God, or Whatever trying to tell me or make me aware of?

If you follow the philosophy that "everything happens for a reason," well, I could not see it. Even though I knew I wanted to heal this diagnosis and be done with it, I had no idea how I was going to do it. I had spent the seventeen early years of my life studying Catholicism, so I was familiar with the concept of faith. Like most who are brought up this way, I conveniently used faith when I needed it, but it was not a daily practice.

Faith wears many faces and the look of it can—and likely, will—change throughout your journey toward living a healed life. You may question the faith you were raised in. You may encounter faiths you'd never considered before. You may reject long-time philosophies you once considered mostly true. But whatever you do, hold on to something endearing and important for you. Establish a central truth for you. Because that faith can get you through the darkest moments.

As I thought about my faith during this time, it was another step on my journey. This time, for no logical reason I was aware of, I had an intense feeling that I would not fall.

The Importance of Creating Spiritual Connection with Others

At the time of first being diagnosed, I felt like I was on a lone island of "wait and see." I had very few people who understood or could digest all that happened to me, including me. I could talk to my then-wife, friends, and parents, but the responses were one of sympathy, as they encouraged me the best way they knew how, I felt alone. At the time, I did not know how to ask for help or receive it. I was in shock and hid it very well. I was in denial, turning inward, hiding my vulnerabilities. I thought I had limited options and when I spoke to anyone, they were either loved ones or doctors. Neither road led anywhere, leaving me in a holding pattern. I knew I needed to get out of this space, and I was open enough to try anything, as long as it was not in a wait-and-see holding pattern.

I made a mental list of what I knew and what I had available outside of doctors and family. I had no idea where to start. If all of this was happening for a "reason," then something—anything—throw me a frickin' bone and let me know where to start. The more lost and alone I felt, the more the avoidance and denial of my diagnosis turned into anger. Anger at myself for the decisions I made in my life, the struggle I was putting my family through, and anything else I could think of at the moment. I turned the holding pattern of "wait and see" into one of anger and blame, exactly what I did not want.

I was looking for work—for anyone hiring—and flailing. I leveraged my network for connections and introductions to job openings. I wanted to provide security for my family and relieve a little of the mounting stress that consumed me. I doubled up my professional demeanor and swept MS and my feelings of not being enough under the rug.

As I continued to read the chapter on MS and the remainder of *Medical Medium*, I saw a little hope and grabbed on tight. I wanted to know why all this was happening, and then, the door to a Dr. Terry Wahls video opened. This led to other talks, philosophies, ideas, doctors. It became an obsession. I explored endless rabbit trails, pursuing books and other media on reversing MS. Some trails were bare in front of me, and others were so apparent—like the awareness of knowing. I had no idea which way I was heading, but I followed how I was feeling and used joy as a barometer to know if I was heading down the right road for me or not.

I continued to study various teachers I encountered. These teachers included Louise Hay, Anthony William, Deepak Chopra, Michael Singer, Dr. Joe Dispenza, Dr. Gregg Braden, Dr. Bruce Lipton, Neale Donald Walsch, Dr. Terry Wahls, and Dr. David Perlmutter. Each of these people became guides on my journey, although I never met them in person. These, and many other, people hold a massive, profound impact on my journey and are a big reason why I have life back. Although I can now see the good in hindsight, at the time, my resistance to receiving was strong, as I fought the ever-present fear, shame, denial, and anger.

Hope & Options

The situation had little hope and few options. Every option or piece of wisdom made my thoughts seem like a mixed bowl of spaghetti. As I went down one path, taking action on what I read or studied, I hit a roadblock and had to switch directions. If I would have given up or quit when the roadblock came, I would not have gotten up again and kept going. During this time, I leaned into my feelings, as I started to meditate. I knew I needed to change, but I did not know where, what, or how.

At times, it felt like I was steering a freighter with a popsicle stick. As I walked this path, there was always a faint light of hope in the distance. I would read a book on spirituality and Belief, leading me to feelings of knowing, and my hope grew. I would leverage this feeling of hope into further action.

Hope leads us down rabbit trails and paths if we are open to looking for them. The willingness to surrender and receive became the challenge. As I continued to take action, I had faith and Belief that I would not fall and that all these trails were leading me to the answers I looked for. This is easier said than done, especially when the world around you is showing you that it is *not* possible.

At the time, I had told only family and close friends (and of course, doctors who specialized in MS). I was not ready to surrender and tell the world that I felt weak and vulnerable. My then-wife and sister-in-law worked hard to find every option for me to explore, including meeting the top MS expert in the country in San Francisco, so I explored the option. I wanted a second medical opinion.

Second Medical Opinions

When I went after second opinions at UCSF medical center, with the top experts in the MS research in the medical community, the solutions and answers were the same. They speculated on the reasons it was happening, and they believed it was an autoimmune condition that caused MS.

Thirty days before my appointment at UCSF, instead of pacing in wait, I began studying what *Medical Medium* said about clean, nutrient-dense foods for healing. Everything discussed in the book led me down rabbit trails I had not heard of or known before, regarding "eating right." The concept of eating right was so esoteric and convoluted by suggestions, and I did not fully understand what the first step was. I was open to exploring the idea that MS is the Epstein-Barr virus, strengthened and perpetuated as it feeds on toxins, capitalizes on stress and a weakened immune system (Bjornevik et al., 2022).

I gave myself thirty days to see if food was medicine. I would study all I could. I also had the mindset that a person could do anything for thirty days. Because I was experimenting with clean, organic fruits and vegetables, what was the harm or danger?

I delved head-first into research on alternative MS cures that controlled the symptoms. I read a story of Dr. Terry Wahls, a clinical professor of medicine at the University of Iowa Carver College of Medicine, who was diagnosed with MS in 2000. Because of her academic medical training, she knew that research in animal models of disease is often twenty or thirty years ahead of clinical practice. She discussed seeking out vitamins and supplements that have been found to help any type of brain disorder, which eventually led her to form The Wahls Diet, which is based around eating what our ancestors ate: a diet that consists of fresh, organic fruit, vegetables, nuts, grass-fed meats, and fish. At the time of starting the diet, she was wheelchair bound and getting worse. A year later, she would be walking without assistance and taking 18-mile bike rides.

I started to see other options, and my hope grew. I just needed the strength and faith to explore them. What was I giving up? A 27 percent chance that I was wrong and I would end up in a wheelchair? (as one doctor alluded too). I liked my odds better on my decisions, and my faith continued to grow; my faith that I would *not* be in the prescribed wheelchair.

Inside physically and mentally, I could feel the difference in my general feeling and demeanor. I used this feeling of hope to build my belief, as I delved head-first into the concept that food is medicine.

This starting point became the basis and reason for me reversing MS and feeling better. That continued action and not giving up when I was discouraged or felt lost led me to gain control that was fueled with hope. My hope was reinforced with my faith and Belief, which led me to a feeling of love and joy for myself.

I knew what I wanted—to heal MS, to eventually walk my daughter down the aisle at her wedding, and to run with my grandkids. I knew Who I Was—a tenacious, never-stop, open-minded, vivacious learner who refused to give up or give excuses. I began to view myself as a badass; this identity was more for me than anyone else. So, when new information and concepts were presented to me, I was open to exploring them. When I had moments when I shook, became dizzy, or my mood shifted—which was often—I could get close to *why* it was happening. Through my newfound education, I could pinpoint a possible cause—food, hydration, or stress—and I had to have faith that what I was exploring was right. Every step gave me hope, as I continued down this path.

Having Faith

Faith can be difficult to embody and live because of the little negative voice mentioned in earlier chapters. If we all have a little negative voice that tells us 80 percent of the time that we are not right, we have the choice whether to listen to it. I knew not to listen to the naysayers, but having the faith and a belief I could do this drowned out the noise. It did not mean I did not listen to everyone's advice, it was how I interpreted the advice and how much weight I gave it that mattered.

Faith, positive thought, and being Who I Wanted to Be was like building muscle. I equated this step like training for Ironman. I needed to be okay in moments that hurt and I could not answer why. This frustration could halt my progress, and the fear of making the wrong choice would leave me in anger. At times, it felt like I did not know what I was doing, and it became a full-time job to keep the imposter syndrome at bay. Just like training for Ironman, I had to have a plan—which included the hope and possibility that I would cross the finish line.

I began to see and experience the importance of faith and Belief to put us out of our comfort zones of possibility. Through all my ups, downs, injuries, and medical challenges, I realized the importance of believing that I would finish, along with the faith that it was already happening. Our intentions and plans can become critical toward the negative voice from others, and more importantly, ourselves.

Like my training plan that helped me obtain the designation of All-American and cross the finish line of Ironman, I developed a plan for healing. This plan became more important than any athletic endeavor or previous desire because it meant my quality of life. It signified whether or not I would live my remaining years bound to a wheelchair.

> You have completed some powerful work throughout this book, and now it is time to take the most critical step: *Your Belief.*

Belief and faith are something you either know or not, but like a muscle, they take time to develop. So, why not have a plan for doing so? My faith plan worked for me, and I encourage you to explore and build your own. Below, I have included my plan—not to be duplicated, but to help you begin a very important step toward your healing.

Chapter 12 Exercise

The Belief Plan

My Belief Plan:

1. Be aware of negative thoughts and ask, "Is this true?"

2. Be curious, as long as it does not have any risk of hurting me or the outcome is negative.

3. Use joy as a barometer: Do I enjoy what I am doing? Am I remaining curious?

4. Meditate. Remember, "The way out is through."

5. Ask for help.

6. Do not let my inner negative voice be in charge. Use it to ask thoughtful questions. Do not allow it to bring me lower.

7. Understand when I am moving too fast and when to slow down

These steps are meant to reinforce and help assist your previous work of identifying Who You Are and What You Want. If you approach your work regarding Who You Are and What You Want with Belief and your faith plan, you will ward off negativity and doubt that inevitably creeps in, closing the door to other possibilities.

We often do not know how we go from point A to point B and can only see the first step. The size of this first step depends on faith and belief in yourself. This faith helps you to keep moving, no matter the adversity. If Thomas Edison did not have Belief, would he have quit trying to make the light bulb work after countless attempts?

The challenges, as in all things, happen when our plan does not work, or when our external reality is different from our desires. Without faith and Belief, we can be tossed around with every setback or struggle, leaving us frozen with no action. Healing is not linear, and at times, we take three steps forward and two back. If we take time to plan, we anticipate these setbacks and slow down to celebrate our wins. We show ourselves that what we are doing is possible, and we are encouraged to keep moving.

When I was training for Ironman and feeling frustration when my leg was not working while running, I would repeat a quote said to me years before: "Failure is not falling down but not getting back up."

> Use your work as the guidepost of possibility and your Belief as the fuel to get back up and keep moving.

Chapter 13

Living without Fear

"Everything you want is on the other side of fear."

– Jack Canfield, *The Success Principles*

Every time I had a TIA episode or stumbled while walking, due to the MS, I felt fear wash over me. Was this going to be the rest of my life? Was I going to die an early death and not be able to see my grandkids someday?

As I thought about these questions, I felt the fear of a reality that had not yet happened wash over me. This deep contemplation of my fear led me to the questions: What do I want? and Who do I want to be?

This deep thought process can set you on a path to let go of the past, not worrying about the future so that you may begin living in the Present Moment. As we think about our fear, we can be overcome with regret, shame, and anxiety about unknown futures. I remember how I felt after experiencing the TIAs and receiving the MS diagnosis; the fear and anger became overwhelming, as I thought about the choices I made and why this happened. At that time, if anyone said, "Everything happens for a reason," I would avoid seeing them again, as the victimhood of my situation washed over me.

These thoughts left me frozen in time and kept me from taking any action or hearing others as they tried to help. What they did not realize was my fear of dying and losing everything; that was the reason I stopped living.

We are not told how we are going to die. We only have an awareness that we are going to die someday. With the absoluteness of this pending situation, we do not discuss death. We treat it as a taboo topic.

Even writing these statements could not be done without experiencing it firsthand, being faced with fear of this reality. It was not until I faced this demon head-on when I was able to release it from my life and begin living a life worth living. As I stepped into this realization, I thought about the choices I was making, and I began thinking about the legacy I would leave for my kids, beyond the monetary legacy—the memories, how they would tell my story when I was no longer there to influence it. Would they remember me as a person of love and joy, or one of anger and fear?

As you think of this topic of fear, make choices that serve you both physically and mentally. When presented with more options and choices—which I know you will be faced with—I want you to think about What You Want, so your choices align with Who You Are and Who You Want to Be.

As I sat on my back deck, alone, facing my fear, I found myself in the peaceful Present Moment. I listened to the songbirds in the tree, the buzz of the bees dancing from flower to flower. I felt the warm autumn breeze. I was reminded that another season was ending, and a new one was emerging. I correlated this flow of life to my own realization that, with every struggle or challenge, is also an opportunity, if we choose to learn and take action with no fear.

As we look at our health challenge as an opportunity, we see the gift. Would you be reading this book right now, on a path of discovering Who You Are, choosing to begin living the life you want?

In the moment of being diagnosed with a disease, we have two roads we can walk down when fear washes over us. We can either choose the path of love and joy, focusing on the Present Moment and living the life we want, or we can remain in fear, living with regret for the life we wished we would have lived. As discussed in earlier chapters, when fear is all-encompassing, we stop looking at the life we want to live. Our minds become closed to a higher level of thinking, and we stew in the past. If we are not careful, the fear can lead to depression and not loving ourselves through a difficult moment, when compassion is required to get through.

Disease as a Burden

I began to think about the burden that I may or may not put my family through. Would they have to push me in a wheelchair, make all of my meals, and someday experience me dying an early death? The fear of death would cross my mind from time to time, but I found myself with the fear of what I may be doing to those I loved. If I circled in the thoughts of being a burden, Who I Was would change into a person I did not want to be. My demeanor would change to one of a victim, declaring that all this was happening *to* me and not *for* me.

Prior to being diagnosed, I noticed obvious changes in my mood. I was regularly angry, frustrated, scared, and depressed, with a general feeling of being lost. I did not understand or know why. I thought it was the stress of my job and helping to raise two kids as they became teenagers. I could not quiet the voice in my head, and when my stress increased by little amounts, I could not handle it and would yell. This was not the man I thought I would be, not the man I wanted to be. This was a red flag. I was acting out of character, but I was not aware of this unwanted change, due to being blinded by fear.

These moments when we are uncomfortable and not our true, authentic Selves can be the wake-up call we need,to stop an undesired pattern of behavior. If you notice a change in your behavior—such as being angry, frustrated, scared, depressed, or another unwanted behavior, with a general feeling of being lost—take a step.

The step I want you to take is an easy first step:
Become aware of these feelings.

Whether you choose to seek outside help—which I highly recommend—the first step is recognizing the behavior, then asking yourself the question: "Am I being my true, authentic Self?"

For me, I felt like a body with an unpredictable angry master at the helm. I wanted to stop and end this angry master who was dictating my thoughts and sense of self-worth. When I was diagnosed—although I did not realize it at the time—I was being forced to face the intolerant, angry master head-on.

This struggle of Who I Was and What I Wanted took time, as I was being led to go within. I slowed down, meditated, and adjusted my diet, all while being open to receiving the teachings of my masters, teachers, and guides. I realized that, yes, I needed to work on myself from a mental aspect but also from a toxin aspect, using food as medicine.

These slow steps and actions I took toward halting MS could not have happened if I had not gone in and found myself. If I had remained in fear, in the victim-state of disease and injuries, I would have remained blind, not seeing that MS was not happening *to* me but *for* me.

Making an Important Choice

As I woke in the morning, the negative voice was the first thing I heard. This voice led to the fear that I was not enough. I could not see myself rising above the disease, gaining the lessons, and taking the actions necessary. I was not looking at the disease as an opportunity to go inside and discover who I was. The actions to not be defined as the disease—which included slowing down, setting loving boundaries, discovering toxins in my food, and ultimately loving myself—was as wide and mysterious as the ocean.

At this moment, I made a choice and began seeing things differently. I made the choice to no longer live in fear. In hindsight, this moment became the starting point to begin taking my life back. As I made this choice, I listened to the quiet, gentle voice of compassion to encourage me forward. I was open to hearing new ways, new thoughts, and new beliefs in order to not be defined by MS or any other challenge.

Belief to Heal

This led me down the thread of toxins in our environment and food. The symptoms from having these toxins in my body was similar to what I faced mentally; for example, I noticed brain fog and an upset stomach after eating gluten. I took the time to study books like *Grain Brain*, by Dr. Perlmutter, to become aware of the effects of gluten on our brains and bodies.

The legacy of Who I Was and Who I Wanted to Be became a driving reason and purpose. I wanted to live a life worth living, and I found this through serving others. Serving others became the purpose of my actions. If I wanted to leave a legacy for my children and grandchildren, I could not be careless, like I had been in the past.

I knew death was on the horizon, as it is for all of us, and I was being forced to address it head-on. Then, I began to notice positive changes and different thoughts. Like a garden that needs to be watered and tended to, I was weeding out the thoughts and actions I did not want and watering and fertilizing the thoughts and actions that brought me love and joy. As I felt better with each passing day, I became curious as to why, which led me down paths of food as medicine, my relationship with God as the creator, and a relationship with myself as the creator of my life.

The choice to face your fear will be the most important step you take on your journey to begin healing mentally and physically. All your fears are real for you. Our fears and the significance we give them are driven by our perceptions of the situations and events in our lives. Your perception will be different than mine. The choice to continue living in this fear is completely up to you.

If you find yourself in a situation where you are trapped, you still have a choice, even if that choice is to do nothing. In times when I feel like I do not have a choice, I am reminded of the story of Viktor Frankl, an Auschwitz survivor during the Nazis' imprisonment and murder of millions of people. His official biography on the website of the Institute that bears his name details everything he went through. Although Victor lost his wife, all his children, and his way of life, he still decided to find light in his terrible situation. He decided to forgive and live from his highest Self, giving to others and finding gratitude from an impossible situation. His way of being allowed him to live in order to influence and help so many people during his imprisonment, and many years after. Through his situation, he still had to make a choice.

> Like you. You have a choice of
> Who You Want to Be and decide which
> lessons you wish to learn from your situation.

Shifting Mindset from "Loss" to "Gift"

As I started to remove toxins, slow down, and meditate, I began to breathe differently, look at events differently; I stopped taking life so seriously. I realized I was trying to control something that needed me to surrender to it. I stopped focusing on the future I was trying too hard to create—which left me with anxiety—and a past that left me with regret and sadness. I began to focus on the Present Moment and thinking about how I was going to live now.

> How did I want to live my life now?
> How was I going to love, serve, and
> release the fear that was stopping me?

I made a conscious choice to deal with all decisions and choices when they arose in the Present Moment. This did not mean I did not plan and prepare for certain choices in the future. I did not allow these plans and choices to become anxiety of the unknown that I could nothing about. Instead, I set the path and dealt with the choices when they arrived.

For example, early on I remember sitting in my neurologist's office, and the topic of treatment came up. After reading all I could about the disease-modifying drugs (DMD) that had a lower success rate than the potential harm they could cause, I became curious (Multiple Sclerosis Trust, 2022). I began looking at all my choices instead of succumbing to a fear there was only one option. I stayed in the moment and listened to how I felt, and I kept the doors of options open.

The flow of life has the answers we are looking for, if we are open to hearing them. This path requires patience, faith, and a belief that what you are doing is right, as you let your intentions of What You Want become the driving force.

As I continued to lean in and remain open to new possibilities, MS became the greatest gift ever handed to me because I woke up to the most important person in my life: *Me*.

For a powerful first step, I would like you to look at the fears that you may be experiencing now.

Chapter 13 Exercise

Write Down all Your Fears

Once these fears are on paper, ask yourself the question, "*Is it true?*" with each fear you have written.

Some may be in your current reality—for example, the fear of not walking, being sick in bed, or something else that feels out of your control—but is this the true reality you desire?

> Who told you that it had to be this way?

As the creator of your own reality, take the time to imagine a new reality for each of these fears. Once you have the new reality in your imagination, how does this new reality *feel*? Whenever your negative past enters your mind with fear, replace it with the new imagined reality, feeling it, as if it already happened.

Try to imagine the new reality of What You Want as a vision in your mind twice per day: once in the morning when you wake up, and again in the evening, before you go to bed.

This starts to create the life, health, wealth, and love that you desire in your life. As you think of these moments, be open to listening and to taking inspired action. As one of my incredible clients says, "If you want to sit in a chair and do not have one and can't go to a store to buy one, you are going to have to make a chair. God gave you the wood of the tree and your hands to build it, but you are going to have to take action to make the chair."

Conclusion

I know you can do this. Be okay with the small steps of progress. The only miracles that arrive in our lives are the ones we Believe in, when we have faith that it has already happened.

As I look at it now, here's what MS did for me:

- Slowed me down.
- Taught me to take a breath before becoming frustrated.
- Made me aware of the dangers of living in the past or future.
- Taught me What I Wanted and Who I Was.
- Inspired laughter.
- Made me aware that vulnerability is strength.
- Showed me how to serve.
- Demonstrated why I must live my Purpose.
- Taught me not to worry about what others think and to focus on what I think about me.
- Provided me with knowledge that I am enough.
- Introduced me to my *Self*.

MS has become a gift, and I am healthier now than I have been in a long time. The cloud of fear that impacted me for all those years has lifted. I am grateful for these moments, and I no longer have any significant thoughts of suicide.

Life's challenges and moments come to us, and we have a choice about how we will treat these moments when they arrive. Death is inevitable, but that is a future I cannot control. Nor do I want to. All I can control are the actions I take now, how I decide to feel, and how to live in the energy of love and joy.

Chapter 14

Inspiring Others

"Do your little bit of good where you are; it's those little bits of good put together that overwhelm the world."

– Desmond Tutu, *Hope and Suffering: Sermons and Speeches*

An Important Lesson Re-Learned: Listening

Six months after I delved head-first into healing MS with food, removing toxins and increasing nutrients, and going within (the start of a spiritual practice), I was referred to a young gentleman who had been recently diagnosed with MS.

I was in the middle of my health coaching certification, felt the best I had in five years, and had a proud understanding and Belief that I was healing. As I spoke to this gentleman, I proceeded to tell him what to do to feel better. I felt it was my responsibility to tell him all I had discovered. *Bad idea.*

That is essentially what I did. My arrogance thought I had the answers. My arrogance thought I knew how to lead him to feeling better. This approach led me to *not* helping him or hearing his struggles from his perspective, which would have truly served him.

Healing MS had been my world, consuming my thoughts for the previous two years. This gentleman was at the start of his journey, and I tried to take him to where I was on my journey. Even though it consumed my thoughts and study, it was not the same for others. I knew this and broke the cardinal rule of having a conversation with anyone: not listening or hearing them.

How was I supposed to assume that I knew how MS was affecting him, what he wanted to do in his life, and what his fears were after being diagnosed? How did I know what help he needed? I could have been someone who listened to his challenges and fears. We all know what "assuming" brings us, and still today, I feel like an ass. The only thing I can do is learn from the interaction and help others by listening and hearing them.

Applying the Re-Learned Lesson

In my past, my superpower was leading and building sales teams. I coached individuals how to listen effectively and seek to understand, before telling or diagnosing. I remember telling the story to those I coached about the analogy of going into the doctor for knee pain.

Imagine the conversation with your doctor goes something like this:

You: Doctor, I have knee pain every time I walk.

Doctor: I have seen this before. It is your ACL. Let's get you scheduled for surgery. I have an opening next week.

If you went into the doctor's office, and the doctor told you what was wrong and went to schedule the surgery before asking you questions or running further tests, you would never go back.

When having a conversation with anyone regarding your approach, reason, or new knowledge, they do not care. Unless they have been with you along your entire journey and thought process, how could you expect to meet them where they are on their own journey? As I studied the best way to approach someone who had been diagnosed with a disease, listening and understanding them became a central theme.

I looked into my own past and remembered the lessons and coaching I gave new professional sales associates. I also remembered the lessons I learned from Donald Miller at StoryBrand.

Lessons from StoryBrand

Do not be the Hero; be the Guide. People do not want to be lectured or told what to do. This approach can lead the individual deeper into fear, or worse, shamed into where they are. For example, the hero in the original *Star Wars* series, Luke Skywalker, did not pursue the path of a Jedi from the beginning. He met Obi-Wan Kenobi who slowly understood Luke's plight and who understood where he was coming from, before introducing or discussing the Force.

It is difficult for people to follow a Hero. They want to follow a *Guide* who goes at their pace and meets them at their level of understanding.

Here are three simple steps to begin leading others as a Guide:

1. Listen so that you hear

People want to be listened to and understood before they can hear you because all our situations are unique. When we first meet someone who may share our challenges, we desire the opportunity to share our unique journey in hopes it will help theirs. It is important to remember at this time that our fears, hopes, and desires are unique to us, based upon our perceptions of our life. When we try to diagnose too quickly or offer advice without understanding fully, we turn off the other individual, and they are more likely to turn away from us than hear our advice, no matter how good it is.

By giving someone the gift of listening, we give our grace and patience. As individuals who may be at the start of a journey and could be riddled with fear, we do not want to hear how someone else may have fixed anything or how someone else did it. As individuals going through the storm of their lives, we desire the opportunity to be understood and listened to.

2. Take your time

Oftentimes, we want to rush because we feel the answer may be easy or urgent. Anytime I rush a conversation, I never feel good about the interaction. I feel like I proverbially vomited all over the individual who just wanted to have a conversation with me. When we step into a realm where something is new, and we are excited about it, we tend to talk more, not less. This most often happens when imposter syndrome ("I have no idea what I am doing") creeps in. Due to this feeling, we want to wow the individual seeking our help with our vast knowledge. Avoid this urge and slow down.

3. Ask questions and be curious

Seek to understand how this diagnosis affects them. Seek to understand how what happened to them may be affecting their life. At times, it will be hard to ask questions, seeking to understand and to be there for someone else. Ask open-ended questions that require more than a "yes" or "no" answer. As the person answers your question and you are listening, pay attention to the vague, fuzzy words that you hear.

For example:

You: Susan, what is taking the majority of your thought and attention right now?

Susan: My kids. I am worried about them.

You: I would like to know more about your worry. Can you tell me more about that?

If you want to help, you should be speaking 20 percent of the time and listening 80 percent.

You will know you are asking the right questions and listening if the other person is relaxed, open to speaking, and wants to do it again. Remember to lean into empathy at this time. Combining empathy and listening will never be wrong.

As I was at this stage in my journey, I often found myself reading Brené Brown (2015) and loved this understanding that she shared: "Empathy is a strange and powerful thing. There is no script. There is no right way or wrong way to do it.

It's simply listening, holding space, withholding judgment, emotionally connecting, and communicating that incredibly healing message of 'You're not alone.'"

For a Reason/Acts of Healing

You received this diagnosis for a reason, and these challenges you face—although very real—are an opportunity to serve someone in need. Just as others appeared and showed up to you at the right time, you can be that for someone else. This act of serving is an important act of healing. The warmth and love you openly give when you help someone feel just a little better, and feeling "not alone" is as much a healing moment for them as it is for you. We all have the opportunity to be there for someone else.

> Sometimes these moments can mean holding the space for them to share. Sometimes these moments can be made of a hug or feeling your love, understanding, and warmth.

There is a reason you are on this journey: Because you have a gift. This gift may show up as listening and being with someone who is experiencing a similar fear to yours. Together, we can go farther and heal as one, using love, empathy, and understanding. With what you have learned, I want to inspire you to pass it forward and help someone else by being the person who can hear them and share their space.

Conclusion

We all have an opportunity, no matter where we are in our own healing journey. This opportunity can be unexpected, and sometimes, it can be from someone who you would not expect it from. We may have a close friend, family member, or a complete stranger who was not diagnosed with the disease but may be experiencing their own fear due to a situation.

We oftentimes do not know why we may have been presented the opportunity to listen to another. When we are presented with this opportunity, we can lean into it or walk away from it; this is a choice, and there is no "right" or "wrong," there just *is*. The damaging thing we can do is judge ourselves or others during this moment.

You are healing and developing your own reasons and beliefs for taking these steps. These moments come as guides for our own journey, even if they are moments of just listening to another. In your journey, you have become a beacon of light that attracts others with your words, your way of being, and more importantly, with your love to hear them. As our mothers told us at a young age, "You have two ears and one mouth, and I hope you use those two powerful appendages that *God* gave you."

Chapter 15

Conclusion

I Believe we are here to learn and understand what our soul desires, and by receiving a diagnosis of any kind, we are given an opportunity to slow down, listen, and know from the depths of our hearts what our soul desires. God, Spirit, Source, or whatever you believe is bigger than all of us—we are one and a part of this oneness with the creator. Our creator is rooted in love, and together, our essence is one of love and compassion. As human beings, we have opportunities to use our gifts, bodies, and souls to uplift others. We are not supposed to walk this journey of life alone. When we hold back and bolt on our masks to be who we are not, we close off the moments of paying attention to how we feel and the inner voice of guidance.

Our world is much greater than what is around you. We are tiny specs in a vast universe that was created just for *You*. You are powerful, and every word you say can go to destroying the beauty around you, or to creating love and grace around you.

> This time, as difficult as it is, will pass,
> and we can take this time to heal or not.
> It is your choice, and that is the great power
> in all of life: your choice and free will.

Take the time to know and understand yourself. Pay attention to the little things around you. Life is giving you answers every minute of every day. It depends on whether or not you want to listen and hear them.

I, along with many others, have our own stories of the guide, guru, teacher, book, or moment happening at the right time, when we needed and were ready to hear their words. We often cannot explain these events in our lives, and we may call them serendipitous or coincidental, as it makes us smile and warms our hearts. These moments are guideposts on our journey, as we continue to take steps forward. Do not take these moments for granted. Look for the love and lesson in each one.

If you are seeking answers, slow down and be open to receiving them. Loosening your grip on life and surrendering can be fearful. When we tighten our grip, it causes anxiety of what may happen in an unknown future. By surrendering and letting go, we are open to receiving. As I have come to understand, nothing can enter a closed hand. Everything wants to see you heal. It is possible, and I challenge you to let go and let it happen.

Yes, you will need to take action on specific steps that are presented to you, like reading this book or following another inspired action that you are led to.

The Belief to Heal came into your life at the perfect time, but it required you to read the first chapter, and then another, and be open to receiving guidance. You can decide to take the steps of discovering Who You Are at the soul level, declaring What You Want, believing that it is already here. You can heal because you are a survivor, and your soul's mission is bigger than a disease.

> No matter what you do after reading this book
> or hearing from another teacher, listen to
> your own guidance from your higher Self.
> There are no "have tos," right or wrong; it just *is*.

There is only your choice, and it is right. You are a guide, and you have been made in the likeness of God, which is rooted in love. You and your soul have a desire to heal, and it is possible, no matter what that means for you. We have to allow it to be, and our life can only create what we desire and Believe.

It is with an open heart of gratitude that I want to thank you for being with me on this journey of rising above your illness as you build and live your Belief to heal. Healing anything in our lives takes practice to develop the muscle of self-love and the encouragement to keep moving forward. I encourage you to find a community either online or locally that hears you and supports your choices. It is easy to stop, but the journey begins when we become curious and are willing to do the work of discovering ourselves.

In love, joy, gratitude, and Belief,

– Matt

If you are interested in joining a group of others who are healing, join the Belief to Heal Facebook Group:

(insert Link)

Sign up for our newsletter to keep up with more encouraging opportunities: www.belief2heal.com

References

Chapter 1

Swindoll, Charles. 2012. *The Grace Awakening: Believing in Grace is One Thing. Living It Is Another.* Thomas Nelson. https://www.amazon.com/Grace-Awakening-Charles-Swindoll/dp/0849911885/ref=tmm_pap_swatch_0?_encoding=UTF8&qid=&sr=

William, Anthony. 2015. *Medical Medium: Secrets Behind Chronic and Mystery Illness and How to Finally Heal.* Hay House. https://www.amazon.com/Medical-Medium-Secrets-Chronic-Mystery/dp/1401948294

Chapter 2

Rumi, Mawlana Jalal-al-Din. n.d. "The Guest House" [poem]. *The Poetry Exchange* website. https://www.thepoetryexchange.co.uk/the-guest-house-by-rumi

Hanh, Thich Nhat. 2012. *Fear: Essential Wisdom for Getting Through the Storm.* HarperOne. https://www.amazon.com/Fear-Essential-Wisdom-Getting-Through/dp/0062004727

Buddha. 1996. *Attavagga: The Self*, verse 165. Translated by Acharya Buddharakkhita. Access to Insight. https://www.accesstoinsight.org/tipitaka/kn/dhp/dhp.12.budd.html

Brown, Michael. 2010. *The Presence Process: A Journey into Present Moment Awareness.* Namaste Publishing. https://www.amazon.com/Presence-Process-Journey-Present-Awareness/dp/1897238460

Singer, Michael A. 2015. *The Surrender Experiment: My Journey into Life's Perfection*. Harmony/Rodale. https://www.amazon.com/Surrender-Experiment-Journey-Lifes-Perfection/dp/080414110X#:~:text=life%20of%20solitude%3F-,Michael%20A.,let%20life%20call%20the%20shots

Ming-Dao, Deng. Multiple references. Explore on Amazon: https://www.amazon.com/Deng-Ming-Dao/e/B000AQ3E0W%3Fref=dbs_a_mng_rwt_scns_share

Brown, Brené. Multiple references. Explore on her website: https://brenebrown.com/books-audio

Dispenza, Joe. Multiple references. Explore on his website: https://drjoedispenza.com/collections

Hay, Louise. Multiple references. Explore on her website: https://www.louisehay.com/products-events/

McEwen, Bruce, as cited in Caldwell, Allison. 2018. "The Neuroscience of Stress." *BrainFacts*. https://www.brainfacts.org/thinking-sensing-and-behaving/emotions-stress-and-anxiety/2018/the-neuroscience-of-stress-061918

Rogers, Carl and Peter Kramer. 1995. *On Becoming a Person: A Therapist's View of Psychotherapy*, 2nd ed. Mariner Books. https://www.amazon.com/Becoming-Person-Therapists-View-Psychotherapy/dp/039575531X

Chandler, Steve. 2005. *Reinventing Yourself: How to Become the Person You've Always Wanted to Be*, 2nd ed. Career Press. https://www.amazon.com/Reinventing-Yourself-Revised-Become-Person/dp/1564148173

Chapter 3

Brown, Brené. 2010. *The Gifts of Imperfection: Let Go of Who You Think You're Supposed to Be and Embrace Who You Are*. Hazelden Publishing. https://www.amazon.com/Gifts-Imperfection-Think-Supposed-Embrace/dp/159285849X

Buddha, as quoted by Bukkyō Dendō Kyōkai. 2005. *The Teachings of Buddha.* Sterling Paperbacks. https://www.amazon.com/Teaching-Buddha-Bukkyo-Dendo-Kyokai-ebook/dp/B00ARH5DZI/ref=tmm_kin_swatch_0?_encoding=UTF8&qid=&sr=

Cohen, Sheldon, as quoted by Carnegie Mellon University. 2012. "Stress on Disease." *Carnegie Mellon University* website. https://www.cmu.edu/homepage/health/2012/spring/stress-on-disease.shtml

Shmerling, Robert. October 27, 2020. "Autoimmune Disease and Stress: Is There a Link?" *Harvard Health Publishing* blog. https://www.health.harvard.edu/blog/autoimmune-disease-and-stress-is-there-a-link-2018071114230

Hemingway, Ernest. 1926. *The Sun Also Rises.* Scribner Publishing. https://www.amazon.com/Sun-Also-Rises-Ernest-Hemingway/dp/0743297334

Chapter 4

Hippocrates, as quoted in Excellence Reporter. 2020. "Hippocrates: On the Wisdom of a Healthy Life." *Excellence Reporter* website. https://excellencereporter.com/2020/10/30/hippocrates-on-the-wisdom-of-a-healthy-life/

Wahls, Terry. Multiple references. Explore on her website: https://terrywahls.com/shop/

William, Anthony. 2015. *Medical Medium: Secrets Behind Chronic and Mystery Illness and How to Finally Heal.* Hay House. https://www.amazon.com/Medical-Medium-Secrets-Chronic-Mystery/dp/1401948294

Cialdini, Robert. 2006. *Influence: The Psychology of Persuasion,* Revised edition. Harper Business. https://www.amazon.com/Influence-Psychology-Persuasion-Robert-Cialdini/dp/006124189X

Chapter 5

Emerson, Ralph Waldo. 2014. *Ralph Waldo Emerson Essays*. A Word to the Wise. https://www.amazon.com/Ralph-Waldo-Emerson-constantly-accomplishment/dp/1783947764

Rogers, Carl, as cited by Saul McLeod. 2014. "Carl Rogers Theory." *Simply Psychology*. https://www.simplypsychology.org/carl-rogers.html

Vujicic, Nick. Multiple references. Explore on his website: https://nickvujicic.com/

Chapter 6

Lao Tzu. (1994). *Tao Te Ching*. Harper Perennial. https://www.amazon.com/Tao-Te-Ching-Laozi/dp/0060812451

Tseng, Julie and Jordan Poppenk. July 13, 2020. "Brain meta-state transitions demarcate thoughts across task contexts exposing the mental noise of trait neuroticism." *Nature Communications* 11, no. 3840. https://doi.org/10.1038/s41467-020-17255-9

Oppong, Thomas. 2017. *One Percent Better: Small Gains, Maximum Results*. https://www.amazon.com/Power-One-Percent-Better-Maximum-ebook/dp/B01N9SZA5I

Cabane, Olivia Fox and Judah Pollack. 2017. *The Net and the Butterfly: The Art and Practice of Breakthrough Thinking*. Portfolio. https://www.amazon.com/Net-Butterfly-Practice-Breakthrough-Thinking/dp/1591847192

Chapter 7

Tolle, Eckhart. 2004. *The Power of Now: A Guide to Spiritual Enlightenment*. New World Library. https://www.amazon.com/Power-Now-Guide-Spiritual-Enlightenment/dp/1577314808

Gladwell, Malcolm. 2011. *Outliers: The Story of Success*. Back Bay Books. https://www.amazon.com/Outliers-Story-Success-Malcolm-Gladwell/dp/0316017930

Sivers, Derek. 2009. "No Yes. Either Hell Yeah! Or No," excerpt from *Anything You Want: 40 Lessons for a New Kind of Entrepreneur*. https://sive.rs/hellyeah

Chapter 8

Gandhi, Mahatma, as quoted in Taro Gold. 2004. *Open Your Mind, Open Your Life: A Book of Eastern Wisdom*. Andrews McMeel Universal. https://www.amazon.com/Open-Your-Mind-Life-Eastern/dp/0740727109

Hoyt, Rick and Dick Hoyt. Multiple references. Explore on their website: https://teamhoyt.com/

Reinertsen, Sarah. Multiple references. Explore on her website: https://www.alwaystri.com/

Chandler, Steve. 2017. *Right Now: Mastering the Beauty of the Present Moment*. Maurice Bassett. https://www.amazon.com/Right-Now-Mastering-Beauty-Present/dp/1600251099

William, Anthony. 2015. *Medical Medium: Secrets Behind Chronic and Mystery Illness and How to Finally Heal*. Hay House. https://www.amazon.com/Medical-Medium-Secrets-Chronic-Mystery/dp/1401948294

Wahls, Terry. Multiple references. Explore on her website: https://terrywahls.com/shop/

Chapter 9

Winfrey, Oprah. 2002. "What Oprah Knows for Sure About Freedom". *O, The Oprah Magazine*. https://www.oprah.com/spirit/what-oprah-knows-for-sure-about-freedom

Chapter 10

Dyer, Wayne. September 3, 2010. "The Ego Illusion." *Wayne Dyer* blog. https://www.drwaynedyer.com/blog/the-ego-illusion/

Chapter 11

LTL Mandarin School. January 3, 2019. "The Most Common Chinese Proverbs, Revealed and Explained." *LTL Mandarin School* website. https://www.ltl-shanghai.com/chinese-proverbs/#chapter-4

Carroll, Lewis. 1991. *Alice's Adventures in Wonderland*. Project Gutenberg. Last modified October 12, 2020. https://www.gutenberg.org/files/11/11-h/11-h.htm

Chapter 12

Saint Augustine. c. 399. "Concerning Faith of Things Not Seen." *New Advent Church* website. https://www.newadvent.org/fathers/1305.htm

William, Anthony. 2015. *Medical Medium: Secrets Behind Chronic and Mystery Illness and How to Finally Heal.* Hay House. https://www.amazon.com/Medical-Medium-Secrets-Chronic-Mystery/dp/1401948294

Chopra, Deepak. Multiple references. Explore on his website: https://www.deepakchopra.com/

Braden, Gregg. Multiple references. Explore on his website: https://www.greggbraden.com/

Lipton, Bruce. Multiple references. Explore on his website: https://www.brucelipton.com/

Walsch, Neale Donald. Multiple references. Explore on his website: http://www.nealedonaldwalsch.com/

Perlmutter, David. Multiple references. Explore on his website: https://www.drperlmutter.com/

Bjornevik, Kjetil, Marianna Cortese, Brian C. Healy, Jens Kuhle, Michael J. Mina, Yumi Leng, Stephen J. Elledge, David W. Niebuhr, Ann I. Scher, Kassandra L. Munger, and Alberto Ascherio. January 13, 2022. "Longitudinal analysis reveals high prevalence of Epstein-Barr virus associated with multiple sclerosis." *Science* 375, no. 6578. 296–301. https://www.science.org/doi/10.1126/science.abj8222

Chapter 13

Canfield, Jack. 2006. *The Success Principles: How to Get from Where You Are to Where You Want to Be.* William Morrow Paperbacks. https://www.amazon.com/Success-Principles-TM-Where-Want/dp/0060594896

Perlmutter, David. 2013. *Grain Brain: The Surprising Truth about Wheat, Carbs, and Sugar—Your Brain's Silent Killers.* Little Brown Spark. https://www.amazon.com/Grain-Brain-Surprising-Sugar-Your-Killers/dp/031623480X

The Viktor E. Frankl Institute of America. n.d. "The Life of Viktor Frankl." *Viktor Frankl Institute of American* website. https://viktorfranklamerica.com/viktor-frankl-bio/

Multiple Sclerosis Trust. March 2022. "Disease Modifying Drugs (DMDs)." *Multiple Sclerosis Trust* website. https://mstrust.org.uk/about-ms/ms-treatments/disease-modifying-drugs-dmds#:~:text=Disease%20modifying%20drugs%20(DMDs)%20are,by%20people%20with%20progressive%20MS.

Chapter 14

Tutu, Desmond. November 1, 1984. *Hope and Suffering: Sermons and Speeches.* Wm. B. Eerdmans Publishing Company. https://www.amazon.com/Hope-suffering-speeches-Desmond-Tutu/dp/0802836143

Miller, Donald. 2022. "StoryBrand: Clarify Your Message." *StoryBrand.* https://storybrand.com/

Brown, Brené. April 7, 2015. *Daring Greatly: How the Courage to Be Vulnerable Transforms the Way We Live, Love, Parent, and Lead.* Avery. https://www.amazon.com/Daring-Greatly-Courage-Vulnerable-Transforms/dp/1592408419

About Author Matt Rowe

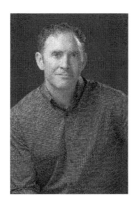

Matthew Rowe, BA, is an All-American Triathlete, Certified Health Coach, meditation practitioner, Reiki master, TEDx speaker, and father of two. In 2010, Matt healed himself from a paralyzed leg to finish the infamous Ironman triathlon, reversed daily activity of TIAs (also known as "mini-strokes"), and recovered from debilitating symptoms of multiple sclerosis (MS) to live his best life. He is the founder of Identity of Health wellness coaching and hosts the Identity of Health podcast. A lover of Self and life, Matt lives in Colorado and travels nationally to speak on Belief, healing, and possibility.

Read more about Matt's journey:

www.mattrowecoaching.com/about

Made in the USA
Middletown, DE
29 October 2024

63507133R00115